Praise for *The Ti*

"In *The Tiger and the Cage*, the call ι̣_ _ _ _ ̦̦̦̩̩ ̦ -
or, rather, from inside the body. In the beautiful prose of a poet,
Emma Bolden confronts the patriarchal foundation of the institutions that make our lives what they are: education, religion, medicine.
If patriarchy—and frankly, misogyny—is part of medical 'care,' then
via each surgeon's scalpel and each prescribed medication, it is also
inside us. *The Tiger and the Cage* opened my eyes, enraged me, and
left me in awe of Bolden's enormous talent as a writer, intelligence as
a critic, and courage as a survivor."

—Maggie Smith, author of *Goldenrod* and *Keep Moving*

"A harrowing portrait of endurance and grief and resilience. With raw
honesty and exacting detail, Bolden tells an intimate story while ex-
ploring the demands our oppressive culture places on women—our
supposed hopes and dreams, our supposed desires and fears, and most
poignantly of all the expectations on our bodies, what they should
do and how they should behave. It is part damning critique of our
male-dominated medical institutions and, quietly, a loving tribute to
a mother-daughter bond."

—Julianna Baggott, author of *The Seventh Book of Wonders*

"Layer by shimmering layer, Emma Bolden transforms the story of
her body into the story of a search for truth. *The Tiger and the Cage*
elegantly interrogates narratives of gender, pain, sexuality, and family
to reveal the freedom underneath."

—Angela Chen, author of *Ace: What Asexuality Reveals About
Desire, Society, and the Meaning of Sex*

"In brief, lyrical, and powerful essays, Emma Bolden unleashes her
story of endometriosis, and the misogyny she endured at the hands

of the medical establishment, interwoven with stories of a supportive and loving Southern upbringing. *The Tiger and the Cage* is a torrent of feeling. It is a left-hook to the jaw to anyone learning for the first time about the neglectful ways women are often treated when their bodies need help. It is a soft, supportive whisper to those of us who know it too well. May it find its way into the hands of doctors and those in training, and their patients, too, who will find a voice in this book, one speaking with clarity and purpose, that affirms their own experiences."   —Chantel Acevedo, author of *The Distant Marvels*

"Emma Bolden's *The Tiger and the Cage* is a memoir written as an investigation, a dive into what it means to be a woman caught in a medical establishment that doesn't listen to women. I read this book in a fury. Bolden's imagery is stark and vivid, and the prose moves in a spiral, encircling her pain, her confusion, and her strength. This book will make you laugh, cry, scream, and bleach your hair while you sing along loudly to Tori Amos. I am so grateful *The Tiger and the Cage* exists and so grateful for Emma Bolden's generosity."
     —Emme Lund, author of *The Boy with a Bird in His Chest*

"This philosophical, funny, and beautiful memoir is both a work of art and a deep conversation about the rift between mind and body, those two great friends and rivals handcuffed together forever. Well-armed with a genuine Greek chorus, a truly excellent and private sense of humor, and incredible gifts for metaphor, Emma Bolden opens the vault for the reader into the true experience of how it feels to both reckon daily with a ravaging illness and also to carry on and make the most of one's life.

"If literature is the great river that runs alongside life, interpreting it, then this book is that river—[it] is deep and vigorous and vital, flashing with transcendence, thinking so richly about the human body, wondering at its mortality and fragility with love and humor and patience and strength."

—Rebecca Lee, author of Bobcat and Other Stories

Praise for *House Is an Enigma*

"*House Is an Enigma* is a staggering achievement. These poems worry several stones in their pockets—grief and the body, certainly, rubbing both until they gleam—but also language and its deliciously endless possibilities. What can I say but that the mind whirring inside these poems, this beautiful lyric-building mind, is one I wish were housed in my own skull? What can I say but give yourself over to these poems, and if you're very, very lucky, some of Emma Bolden's genius may seep into you—and leave you, too, irrevocably changed."

—Maggie Smith, author of Good Bones

"Emma Bolden's gorgeous poems brilliantly remind me of learning to draw with colored pencils. To make a pencil drawing really stand out, one must begin with the lightest of touches and unexpected colors, like, say, lavender—for a banana. Her poems ache with intelligence while layering desire, melancholy, and a delicate grief—and before you know it, we are transported to years where 'we wore leather & guitar music sweet with distortion' and savored 'the taste of peppermint bright as teeth.' Bolden's poems are visceral and profoundly precise—all while balancing a quiet playfulness and dazzle of color that I know I'll return to again and again."

—Aimee Nezhukumatathil, author of Oceanic

"Emma Bolden writes: 'House doesn't care about your intentions, your repairs. House dares / you.' Every poem in *House Is an Enigma* is a dare—a window opening to a gorgeous room or century, a terrifying or luminous sky. It is also a brilliant, inventive, and deeply felt exploration of loss—namely, the potential for motherhood and all that future-imagining might entail. Filled with ghosts, skywriters, skulls, mouths, and fragile crinoline beauty, these poems dwell in the liminal space of self-questioning and what it means to inhabit an imperfect female body. Can one separate the body's lost creative potential from language itself? What are we without our imagining? If the poet is cut off from the metaphor of the body as a home/house, what is there? But Bolden's questioning is not devoid of life, love, or longing—quite the opposite. Please open yourself to Bolden's witchy, wise, and breathtaking vision—what's possible for all of us in the long hallways of our hearts."

—Sarah Messer, author of *Dress Made of Mice*

"Emma Bolden's *House Is an Enigma* is a masterful book that serves as a map through the dark museum of loss. 'After great pain, a formal feeling comes,' Emily Dickinson writes, and Emma Bolden's poems are the light that we, as readers, will 'wonder out towards' after the formal feeling has gone: 'Let grief be the song that troubles down / the keys of your spine.' The music that emanates from these poems can fill even the largest room that loss can build. These poems boldly become light even in the face of the darkest of darks."

—Adam Clay, author of *Stranger*

THE TIGER AND THE CAGE

ALSO BY EMMA BOLDEN

House Is an Enigma
medi(t)ations
Maleficae

THE TIGER AND THE CAGE

A Memoir of a Body in Crisis

EMMA BOLDEN

Soft Skull
New York

First Soft Skull Press edition: 2022

Grateful acknowledgment for reprinting materials
is made to the following:
Material from: Batt, Ronald E. *A History of Endometriosis*. London:
Springer-Verlag, 2011 reproduced with permission of SNCSC.

Quotes from the Mayo Clinic in chapter 116 used with permission of Mayo
Foundation for Medical Education and Research, all rights reserved.

Library of Congress Cataloging-in-Publication Data
Names: Bolden, Emma, author.
Title: The tiger and the cage : a memoir of a body in crisis / Emma Bolden.
Description: First Soft Skull Press edition. | New York : Soft Skull, 2022. |
Includes bibliographical references.
Identifiers: LCCN 2021060600 | ISBN 9781593767235 (paperback) |
ISBN 9781593767242 (ebook)
Subjects: LCSH: Bolden, Emma—Health. | Endometriosis—Patients—
United States—Biography. | Women poets, American—Biography.
| Asexual people—United States—Biography. | Endometriosis—
Treatment—United States. | Medical personnel—Malpractice—
United States. | Discrimination in medical care—United States. |
Sex discrimination against women—United States.
Classification: LCC RG483.E53 B65 2022 | DDC 618.1/42—dc23
/eng/20220504
LC record available at https://lccn.loc.gov/2021060600

Cover design by Nicole Caputo
Cover art © Bridgeman Images / Young orphan in the cemetery by
Ferdinand Victor Eugene Delacroix
Book design by Wah-Ming Chang

Published by Soft Skull Press
New York, NY
www.softskull.com

Printed in the United States of America

1 3 5 7 9 10 8 6 4 2

For my parents,
with all my love and all my gratitude
for taking every step along with me

He feels as though there were a thousand bars
and behind the thousand bars no world.

RAINER MARIA RILKE
"The Panther"
(trans. Brigitte Wallinger-Schorn)

Contents

PRECIPITATION

1

In fifth grade, my teacher spent an entire semester on the water cycle. I learned how temperatures fall, how water molecules join hands and then jump from the clouds. I learned how, in high clouds, crystal hexagons form. At lower altitudes, water freezes to needles. I learned that the clouds themselves aren't solid structures. Instead, they're collections of microscopic water droplets clinging to dust, to tiny scraps of the earth on which we walk and write in the margins of books and lay down against crisp sheets to sleep. If the temperature falls far enough, ice crystals cluster around dust particles, gathering together into snowflakes brittle enough to break as they fall. In Alabama, snow was a miracle, a tall tale parents told while gathered around an unlit fireplace.

Every night that fall and winter, I watched the weather report and wished for a hard freeze, at least. I chanted the number my teacher told us was the freezing point of water—*thirty-two, thirty-two, thirty-two*—as though it were magic. Incantation. Prayer. On cold days I played a game with the air, holding breath in my lungs until it burst out by its own volition and hung white in the air, an apparition, a sign.

Each night my mother pulled the bedspread to my chin. Each night sleep pulled my lids shut and I pulled against it, trying to stay awake so I could pray—*thirty-two, thirty-two, please God, snow school away*. Sometimes I slipped from my bed to touch my window, checking to see if it felt like freezing, if the line of mercury in the thermometer had finally fallen.

At school, I learned that snowflakes grew into hexagons because they had to. Nature made them that way. When water freezes around a seed of dust, it creates an ice crystal, six arms branching out from the center, water molecules sliding into patterns created by the cloud's conditions. Then more crystals form, branching identically off of the six arms, more molecules following their patterns. It was a reflection of God's great design, my fifth-grade teacher said; the way of a world God created through a series of patterns that endlessly grew and branched off, that swirled backward to repeat. Our own bodies formed under the same kind of artistry, cells gathering and growing into branching patterns: arteries that split into arterioles that split into capillaries, bronchial tubes in the lungs that break into smaller tubes capped with alveoli. If I held the back of my hand close enough to my eye, I could see the lines etched into my knuckles, which traveled and branched out into designs that stayed in place, unlike any snow I'd ever seen.

2

SOME DAYS BEFORE LUNCH MY REGULAR TEACHER WOULD leave, and in her place came the catechism teacher who taught us about miracles, like the priest who doubted the truth of transubstantiation. One morning mass, the catechism teacher told us, he recited the words of Consecration and found the Host had turned to real flesh in his hand, limp and body-warm. In the chalice, wine thickened, acrid as blood. The Vatican later agreed to let scientists test the Host and the wine, our catechism teacher said. On slides, it showed up as cardiac tissue. The wine was blood, type AB, the same as the blood on the Shroud of Turin. She stood at the front of the classroom, eyes closed in blissful prayer, and so she didn't see Timothy Blockner put his finger in his mouth, pointing at his throat while pretending to retch. After that class, we fifth graders walked straight past the line for Communion wine during Friday morning mass.

One winter Friday, our catechism teacher passed out small plastic bags. Inside them were scapulars, small scenes printed on scraps of brown cloth: on one side, a picture of Mary holding the infant Jesus along with her promise: "Whosoever dies clothed in this scapular shall not suffer eternal fire." On the other side, a picture of her heart and Christ's heart joined together by a crown of thorns, pierced through with flaming swords. The catechism teacher told us about a cheerleader who survived a car crash with an eighteen-wheeler, which, needless to say, should've killed her. The paramedics cut off her clothes and found a ribbon arced over her ribs, the two squares of her scapular pinned to the inside of each cup of her bra.

"Wear your scapular at all times, kids," she told us. "If you do die while you're wearing it, you'll go straight to heaven. Otherwise, you'll go to purgatory to atone for your sins."

"That's a bunch of crap," my mother said when I told her. "That woman is one of those weird Catholics. A fanatic. I ought to call the school."

3

When I wasn't wearing my uniform, I liked to wear my favorite shirt, the one with four cats on the front and the same four cats on the back. The front of the shirt showed the fronts of the cats; the back showed their backs. Their tails periscoped upward in a friendly hello kind of way. I wore that shirt the day I walked down the stairs and into the kitchen and my mother said, "Oh," and then, "Emily, you need a bra. I'm sorry, but you do." It was the first time she or anyone else had said that, at least to me, and she said it in earshot of my father. So I said, "Don't say that in front of my *father*," crossed my arms, and marched back upstairs.

When I think of that moment now, I'm embarrassed not because my mother told me and within earshot of my father that I needed a bra but because I was wearing a shirt that featured four cats exposing their indeterminate genitalia, though, at the time, I hadn't yet learned what those exposed parts might mean.

I had learned that humans and cats and dogs and all the mammals that furred and birthed and nursed their young had similarly patterned genitalia. I knew that differences in these patterns indicated whether or not a person or a cat or any mammal was considered a male or a female at birth. I understood, in a theoretical way, that these mammalian parts had something to do with becoming an adult, with making babies, with walking down the humiliatingly pink feminine products aisle at Food World. I just didn't know the exact whats or whys.

No one—not my mother nor my pediatrician nor the gym teacher who told us what deodorant was and why we needed our parents to buy us some immediately—had fully and completely explained periods to me. I'd learned the basics in the waiting room of the doctor my mother saw for her painful periods, where I ate the heads off of clown-shaped cookies and waited for her appointments to end. The pamphlets in the waiting room told me that periods were actually called menses, and everything associated with periods/menses— bleeding, clotting, pain—sounded like a catechism lesson, like a disease that could be cured through the mercy of Mary's sacred heart.

I'd read until I felt too nauseated, as if all the clowns' heads in my stomach were shaking themselves at once in one collective *nope*. Then I'd look at the pictures, which were as difficult to understand as the diagrams that tried to explain aquifers in my science book. The pamphlets showed two landmasses that must've been legs. Between them sat a pink tube, which widened to a pinker triangle that the pamphlet called a uterus. There, one might find a contraceptive device, a tumor, or a baby. I understood that, like the women on the pamphlets, I too had been born with female organs. I understood that the same tubes and triangle floated inside of me.

4

IN THE UPPER CORNER OF EVERY PAGE IN MY SCIENCE BOOK, I drew the shape of a snowflake, each holding out six identically shaped arms, each in erasable blue ink and in a slightly lower position. When I flipped through the pages of the book, snow fell down the margins. Our teacher showed us microscope slides when we didn't believe what she told us about snow. I looked through the lens and there it was, the truth. Though every snowflake stretched out six arms, no two were exactly the same. My teacher's hand trailed chalk across the board. Her breath smelled like mint and onion, sour and milk. It brought goose bumps up on my arms, but she was also the first person to tell me that I was a good writer, to encourage me to write more and more, to tell me she was thrilled to read anything, anything I wrote, to promise without prompting to not show it to or talk about it with anyone. During silent reading time every morning, I wrote instead, then asked for permission to go to the bathroom. Every time, I left a four-times-folded note on her desk. Every time, my cheeks were heat. I felt the strangeness of my knees. I didn't know if it was because I felt embarrassed or because I'd given her another secret. I forgot the strangeness and embarrassment when she gave me a compliment in exchange.

The secrets I gave my teacher were small stories, small gifts: how I'd tried for weeks to lose my first tooth, only to have the dentist excise it, its root overgrown in eruption. How jealous I was of the lipstick-and-blush girls who traded secrets about kissing between bathroom stalls. How sometimes I stared out the window from the passenger seat and wondered what would happen if I opened the door, jumped out onto the road, and then walked all the way home, how sometimes a long road looked like a challenge that had to be wandered alone. While the boys curled loose-leaf into spitballs then loaded their sipping-straw guns, while the girls pretended to read the science book that I used to find questions to ask our teacher—prairie dogs and aquifers, chlorophyll and stratosphere—I carved each secret word of each story with my erasable pen, blue ink smelling faintly of berries, eraser staining the page a light gray. As fall grayed into winter, the boys grew less patient. They folded paper footballs to shoot through a goal made of thumbs and outstretched fingers.

5

WHEN I SLID INTO THE PASSENGER SEAT OF HER BIG burgundy Buick at carpool, my mother asked me to tell her about my day. For a while I tried to roll my eyes in a way that the TV suggested was appropriate for a girl approaching middle school. Then she told me she'd ground me for so long I'd wish my eyes just rolled out of my head. I didn't roll my eyes after that. "Fine, I guess," I'd say. Sometimes she'd roll her eyes and I'd bite my tongue to keep from saying that if I couldn't roll my eyes, she shouldn't be able to either. Then I'd give in, and launch into a recitation of what we learned that day. I told her about aqueducts, how the Romans made them out of volcanic cement, how beavers used branches and twigs to turn a stream their way.

Sometimes we drove straight to her doctor's office, where she brought her body for another appointment. A nurse called her name and she followed her, leaving me in the waiting room next to a lamp with a burning-out bulb. It blinked at me. When the light wasn't blinking, it lit the illustrations on the pamphlets' covers, pink and inscrutable. I tried to focus on my math homework. I hated word problems the most. In their stories, people were always boarding trains at certain times and at certain speeds, but they were bad travelers who never knew when they'd arrive, pass one another, or meet. I stared so intently at the sketches of Train A and Train B that they seemed to lose their train shape and become just lines, just speed.

•

During emergency drills at school, we rushed into the middle school hallway, searching for the student assigned to hold our left hands as we walked between classes, to the playground, to the church parking lot. When an alarm sang one long note, it meant fire. Three staccato notes meant a tornado was following us as we ran to the windowless side of the gym or the hallway that stretched from classrooms to cafeteria. During tornado drills, I sat a careful inch away from my left-hand partner, the blond boy who once called me shitface, who called me a baby for holding our teacher's hand.

We pulled our knees to our chests, put our heads down against them, then circled our arms around our bodies for protection. I froze my body the way I did in playground games that required a self as stiff as the monkey bars, as the swing set's frame. I imagined my arms as icicles, sharp and unmovable, careful not to touch the boy whose quiet breath made a tune about me and our teacher, sitting in a tree. I imagined my arms as tree limbs, thick and straight against wind, against rain. My teacher crossed my name off her roll with the pencil I sharpened for her each morning, now whittled down to an inch. I prayed for the mercy of the Virgin Mary, just in case it wasn't really a drill. I closed my eyes. I was a spine. I was the body inside of my body, the good, strong white only vitamins could touch.

6

I LIKED TO SIT WITH MY LEGS CROSSED, THE WAY THAT THE teachers did in the lunchroom, sipping Diet Coke out of cans and watching to make sure no one threw bologna at anyone's face or on the floor. In the classroom, I could feel my fifth-grade teacher as she walked by, even if I wasn't looking. If my legs were crossed, she'd spread the fingers of her right hand and then close them together on my knee. She'd lift my leg from the other leg and move it until my foot found the floor. "Spider veins," she whispered, like a secret, and then, "You'll thank me later. I promise."

According to our catechism teacher, if you were very holy, sometimes you'd look up at the sky and see the Virgin Mary spinning the sun. That's what happened to Sister Lúcia of Fátima. She looked up and saw the sun spin above her. The Virgin herself said she'd be saved from sin by sacrifice, so Lúcia tied a cord tighter and tighter around her waist, then whipped herself with stinging nettles, taking the pain as a sacrifice for sinners, taking the pain for all those she had been called to heal and save. Because Lúcia had obeyed her, Mary appeared to her in apparitions, giving Lúcia three secrets: three stories, a series of patterns that would, under the right conditions, turn into truth. One was a vision of hell, one a vision of two world wars that branched off of each other, etching their lines across the globe. The third was a vision so frightening that the Virgin Mary asked Lúcia to keep it to herself.

Mary also told Lúcia that women were sinful, that even then

women dressed in ways that would damn them—long, uncovered falls of hair, ankles bare and exposed. The catechism teacher said we all surely shamed Mary now, knees knobbing beneath our short skirts, our elbows bent and plain. How could we expect her to help us?

"That's a bunch of crap," I imagined my mother saying, but I never told her that part of what the catechism teacher said. A secret was a kind of sacrifice. Sister Lúcia kept her secrets unto death, and neither gold coins nor silk dresses could loose it from her lips. Good girls keep quiet, letting others tell their stories. Good girls hold their truths unto death.

7

ONE MORNING, I WOKE IN THE STILL-DARK AND FELT HEAVY everywhere. My feet didn't feel like my feet. I pushed my body out of bed and walked it to the bathroom. And there it was: a spot of blood, sitting in the middle of my panties. There was a spot of blood in the middle of my toilet paper, too, unmistakable and bright. I looked at it for a while before I decided to pretend that nothing was happening. I flushed the toilet paper and washed my hands and went back to bed to panic.

I'd become one of the women in the pamphlets in the waiting room who walked around with all those pink shapes inside of them, cramping and bleeding, doubled over in pain. My throat closed in panic, so I told myself, *Stop thinking about it, stop thinking about it.* I thought it so many times that the words became hollow bells of sound. I realized that telling myself not to think about it was another way of thinking about it.

I pulled the comforter over my head and thought about how stupid *Are You There God? It's Me, Margaret.* was. She'd waited for her period for years, scanning her underwear, searching her body for buds of breasts or blooms of hard, curly hair. Margaret felt like a period was a spectacularly lucky thing to find, like a perfect six-armed snowflake that stayed without melting on a gloved fingertip. I just felt my body between the sheets and the pain inside of my body. It felt so spectacularly unlucky that I decided I must have misread the book.

I sat in the closet and skipped to the chapter when Margaret got

her period. I managed not to cry—until I read about the pink sanitary belt Margaret used to hold up her Kotex. I imagined my waist
looped by thin pink belts. I imagined the wide bed of a Kotex settled
in the crotch of my panties. I cringed at the word *crotch*. I imagined
standing in the hallway before gym class, where all the girls stripped
off our uniform pinafores to reveal the shorts we wore underneath.
There would be pointing. There would be laughing.

For Are-You-There-God Margaret, getting her period meant she
was a woman now, not a little girl, which meant *I* was a woman now,
not a little girl. I thought of the card my father had just given me for
my birthday, with its daisies and the pink girlish script. I thought
of our Saturday library trips, where I followed him through the poetry section, memorizing the spines of every book he touched: Byron,
Cummings, Eliot. We sang Simon & Garfunkel songs on the way
home, making boxing jabs at the dashboard after every *lie la lie*.

I began to get serious about crying. I moved my body to my
mother's bedroom door. She was a breathing lump under the comforter, so I called out for her—"Mom? Mom," and then "Mama" for
good measure. The lump in the comforter made a noise that might've
been a word. It sounded like *what* or *wind* or *whack*.

"I think something's wrong," I said, even though it was a lie. I
didn't have to think.

She rustled out of sleep. Then an arm reached out from under her
comforter to pat the bedside table for her glasses. "What?"

"I think something's wrong." My voice came out squeaking, the
way it did the time I fell off my bike and saw a rock sticking out of a
hole in my knee. "There's blood."

She blurred into action, putting on her glasses, throwing off the
covers, and then throwing her feet over the side of the bed in one
swift motion. "There's blood? Where? What happened?"

"In my panties." I wasn't even speaking anymore. I was wailing.

"Oh," she said, and then a longer *oh*, a drawn-out *oh*, the kind of *oh* she used when I wore the green velvet dress that made her say I was growing up so fast.

Then my mother was out of the bed and next to me. "Baby, it's okay," she said, pulling my face to her chest. I could smell perfume and sweat and baby-powder-scented deodorant, and then my whole body was made of sound, heaving against her chest.

"It's just your period, Peanut." She rocked me back and forth. "You started your period. You're a little woman now." I pressed my face into her nightgown, shaking it back and forth to wipe my face and to say what I wanted to say: *no* and *no* and *no.*

8

I TOLD SAMANTHA LEE THAT I HAD PAJAMAS FROM VICTORIA'S Secret. They were actually a hand-me-down from my mother and also the least Victoria's Secret–like pajamas Victoria's Secret sold: an oversize purple nightshirt with matching purple pants. I did not offer these clarifying details. Samantha Lee raised her eyebrows and said, "Whoa," only she made it into a five-syllable word, more like "whoa-o-o-o-oa." I nodded in what I hoped looked like mysterious wisdom. It felt important to impress her. Samantha was the self-professed playground expert on the female reproductive system and everything it did and might do, including have sex and get a period. Despite the fact that she hadn't yet started her own period, she still sermoned from the small mount of grass behind the stairs to the gymnasium, preaching about Kotex pads flooding with rivered blood, about the girl whose tampon went up too far and ended up in her throat, where it choked her.

Here are some of the things Samantha Lee told me and the other girls in my grade about periods:

If you try to bake when you're on your period, you'll curdle the eggs and ruin the cake.

If you run laps or lift weights while you're on your period, you'll lose calcium so fast it'll honeycomb your bones with holes.

Having a period makes you shark bait and bear bait and snake bait.

Having a period loosens braces and fillings from the semicircle of teeth jeweling your mouth.

Having a period makes you unclean. If you receive the Lord Jesus in Holy Communion while you are bleeding, the Host itself will turn to blood in your mouth.

If your fingers touch its petals while you're having your period, a flower will wither, wilt, and die.

If you take a bath while you have a period, your blood will stop flowing and you'll die.

If you have sexual intercourse during your period, your sexual partner will die.

If you perm your hair during your period, you'll sizzle your hair to the scalp.

If you have a period and use a tampon, you are no longer a virgin.

9

ANYTHING, ANYONE COULD BE CURED, MY FIFTH-GRADE teacher taught us, if they just believed: babies the size of her notecard case survived heart surgery, performed by instruments so small as to be impossible, though nothing, she said, was impossible, so long as we believed. And if we believed, she said, we could breathe water, which was full of oxygen, which our lungs could absorb if we told ourselves they could. In my notes, I told her I was a ghost already. I told her I wondered sometimes if I were asleep, if I just dreamed I was walking around on the world. I told her there were times I wished I'd already left my body behind.

From my teacher, I learned that precipitation refers to any of the things that, by will of nature or design or God, fall from the sky onto the ground. It could mean snow or hail. It could mean rain or mist. It could mean the water that remained, stretching itself over the earth's surface, waiting to evaporate and become cloud again.

From the dictionary, I learned that *precipitate* can mean "to throw violently." To bring about a change, some new state of being. Too abruptly, too suddenly. Too early. Before anyone has had a proper chance to prepare.

My mother showed me how to pull up the plunger to stop the sink's drain. She told me to fill the sink with cold water, holding my red-spotted underwear under the faucet, then letting them soak in the basin.

"You'll need to know how to do this," she said. "The washing machine won't get out all the stains and I am *not* buying new panties every month."

I wondered exactly how much blood I would be losing. I wondered if the pamphlets lied and having a period was actually a disease. I wondered if I would ever stop wanting to barf when I heard the word *panties.*

"Sometimes you'll need to soak them two or three times," my mother said, walking in front of me to my bedroom. She showed me how to find the right pair for periods, fumbling through my drawer past the pairs with the tiny rosebuds that came in perfect packs of pastel threes. She pulled out a pair of plain white Hanes, the kind she bought in six-packs for three dollars. "You need to wear old ones, just in case," she said. Then we walked in solemn procession back to her bathroom. I wondered: *Just in case what?*

I sat on the toilet with my panties stretched between my knees. My mother unwrapped the pink Kotex package and pulled the thin tongue of paper off the pad's back. When she pressed it onto the crotch of my underwear, I'd already steeled myself. I barely blinked when I thought the word *crotch.*

"Make sure it sticks all the way or you'll have an accident, and you don't want that." I pictured the segments that always seemed to open our local news, cars smashing their heads against a bridge's guardrails, spitting their people into the Cahaba River below.

At lunchtime, my mother set the table: three glasses of iced tea, three plates full of pasta salad, all circled around a chocolate cake. On top of the cake, in pink icing, was the word *congratulations* followed by a period. My father drove forty-five minutes from the Buick dealership where he worked as an accountant. He sang his *hello hello* song and kissed us both on the forehead. He'd stopped somewhere to buy a single pink carnation on his way home for lunch. It was the first thing I saw when he walked in the door. The second thing I saw was his face, looking back at me and crumpling immediately into tears, which meant that I immediately crumpled into tears as well. My mother said, "For Christ's sake," and my father hugged me.

"Hey, kid," he said, which was what he always said, which made me cry even harder. We stood together and kind-of-cried and he sniffed and I sniffed until we both laughed. We were ridiculous. My mother told us both to blow our noses.

"I don't know why you were so afraid of growing up," she told me, years later. "It's not like we were going to kick you out or make you pay rent."

The day that I started my period, I sat with my palms flat against the surface of my bathwater. I told myself to remember what my teacher told me. What she told us. "Anything's possible," she'd said, if you believed. One day, she said, we'd all live underwater, breathing the water, like in the movie *The Abyss*. And I could see it, real as television: whole colonies of wanderers fed up with the surface who, one day, took to breathing water, tending their domed houses and eating fish and algae, long-haired kelp. Believe, my teacher said, and the impossible becomes possible, the possible becomes actual.

10

ON MY FALL SEMESTER EXAM, I'D DRAWN WHAT MY FIFTH-grade teacher asked of me, doing my best to copy exactly the drawing she'd made on the board: a cloud made up of six interlocked *C*s, like the half circles that held her mouth in the grimace she'd soften only for me, and then the threads of rain from which hung the sea, a line suspended. Her right hand took my completed test. And my hand. I felt her warmth and the slick of her lotion. I smelled lavender and antiseptic mouthwash. She held the paper and scratched her ribs. I imagined them as skeleton bare, like the ones in our science book, swelling and sinking beneath her turtleneck, the plaid fabric apple stitched over her heart. While her eyes were looking at my eyes, I saw water. I saw the blue I'd seen at the pool's bottom when I felt brave enough to open my eyes, the chlorinated kind of blue that sticks and stings and pricks your eyes red-threaded for the rest of the day. When her eyes slid away to my paper, she half-smiled, her hand still against mine, its thumb moving slowly.

"A natural forger," she half-whispered, her thumb now shifting so the nail slid its curved blade into my palm. Then it was over, my hand free, the test in the out tray. On my palm, a half circle cut out in red. It stung, so I held it against my lips and tasted lotion, perfume and paste, milk unthawed and gone wrong.

11

MY FIFTH-GRADE TEACHER WAS MY FAVORITE BECAUSE SHE listened. She believed. She didn't think of me as my acne or glasses or braces. She told me that I should be myself simply because my self was a very good person to be. She told me she couldn't wait to buy my books someday. In my notes, I told her I didn't know how to talk to my mother anymore, that suddenly she felt like a stranger who yelled at me for forgetting to clean my room and singing too loudly in church, because I acted like the tiniest thing—a pimple, a stomachache—was the end of the world when, I couldn't help but think, anything *could* be the beginning of the end, at least. I told her that I wished I could be like Louisa, with her perfect skin and her perfect vision and her perfect single-file line of teeth. I told her I felt like no one really knew me. I didn't even know myself. I was like an onion or a woman wearing veil after veil.

She vanished just after we returned from Christmas break. I'd spent December in our unused dining room, the blinds quarter-closed to keep in the heat. My mother hummed and washed dishes in the kitchen. I sat at the glass table and put together a puzzle: a picture of the ocean, blue as a sky interrupted by fish. I held my tongue like a secret.

One day after school, I'd stood in the yellow square outside of our classroom, waiting for my mother's Buick to float its way through the carpool line like an embarrassing boat. I felt my teacher's hand on my shoulder. She leaned down and whispered in my ear.

"I'd like to have you visit my house over Christmas break," she said. I smelled the sour in her breath, somewhere under its mint. I smiled and I nodded my head. "I'll call your mother to ask."

When my teacher finally called, my mother walked the phone into her bedroom, closing the door on its extra-long cord. I could only hear murmurs that suggested words, but I understood the gist of the conversation: *Thank you, that's very kind, but we've got so much to do, I'm grateful that you asked, but no.* When she'd said goodbye, my mother walked the phone back to the kitchen. I heard her put the handset back into the base with a clanging finality. She walked into the dining room, rolling her eyes. "That woman could talk the ears off a goat," she said. Then she looked down at me, eyebrows raised and pushed toward each other in an expression I recognized as concern.

"Peanut, I told her you couldn't go to her house. I know you might be disappointed, and I'm sorry. But something just doesn't feel right." Though she hadn't asked a question, I knew my mother wanted an answer, so I nodded. I didn't look at her. "Do you hate me?"

I sat for a moment and asked myself: Did I hate her? Then I shook my head. She was right: I was disappointed, but something just didn't feel right. I just didn't know how to admit that to myself, and I definitely didn't know how to admit it to her. I didn't speak. I heard my mother's footsteps come closer to me, felt her lean down and kiss me on the top of the head.

I didn't know how to talk to my teacher when she came back. I didn't know how I should explain it in a note, the fact that I didn't visit her over the break, the fact that, in some way, it felt like a relief. So I didn't mention it, and in a few weeks, she was gone. I couldn't help but feel guilty. I couldn't help but feel like I'd lost it, my chance to explain.

12

ALL THROUGH THE HOLIDAYS, MY MOTHER STAYED IN THE kitchen, cooking up her cures: chicken soup, mashed potatoes, my favorite cookies coated in icing food-colored to shades of petal and leaf. When she asked what I was thinking, I told her nothing. My mother offered peeled oranges, milk tinged with coffee. Her voice hushed itself on the phone.

A therapist asks me about what happened when I was in fifth grade. She wants to know what I remember. I tell her that I remember my teacher telling me that she was leaving. I stop. I think. I tell her, "Wait, that's not right. She didn't tell me." Instead, I found out from Louisa, the popular girl who smelled of her mother's Chanel, who painted pink circles on her cheeks after being dropped off at school. I was in the cafeteria, sitting uncomfortably and staring down the room's long stretch of tables and bench seats at her bright cheeks. I heard but didn't quite understand the words circling away from her lip-glossed mouth: "She's leaving. She told me. She didn't tell you?"

I felt myself in my body. Boiling. I wondered how I'd respond. To my surprise, I did not cry.

"Why did you say you found out from your teacher at first?" my therapist asks.

"I don't know," I say. "Maybe that's just what I want to believe."

I tell my therapist that I remember seeing my teacher's empty chair, her top drawer emptied of the notes I gave her each day. She'd left them behind. The principal found them. He told my mother he would give them to her. My mother at first refused for my privacy, then, haltingly, asked the principal: "What do I need to know?"

When I found out that my teacher was leaving, I did not cry. I did not cry.

I coughed.

13

AFTER MY TEACHER LEFT, I DREAMED AND I DREAMED. EACH dream was the same. There was a blackboard, and on it a chalked cloud trailed by comma-shaped rain. The rain fell, like stop-motion, slower and slower. When I awoke, the blank was in my throat. My mouth split and it escaped—a cough, and then another cough. The coughs came faster, then faster.

The doctor told my mother to sit me in the shower so its steam would open my throat. She led me into her bathroom's small cubicle and held me up so I could stand and breathe in the steam. I coughed. My chest heaved, the two lobes of my lungs spasmed toward breath. Sometimes I prayed that I'd stop coughing. Sometimes I prayed that I'd never stop coughing. I thought about all the things my teacher told me to believe. Anyone could be cured. Anyone who wanted to be.

There were cough syrups, thick and red as liquid jewels poured precisely to the top line in small plastic cups. There were cherry throat lozenges that tasted like candy kept in a hot car too long. There were inhalers and anti-inflammatories the size of bad beetles. Sometimes I couldn't swallow all the way and my throat pushed the pills back up. I tasted them like bitters on the back of my tongue, a taste that outlasted the Diet Cokes, the ginger ales, the orange sodas meant to bubble and burst my cough. During the day, I watched science programs on public television. Once, I turned on the TV and saw a fox. At first, I thought it was peacefully asleep. Then I realized. The fox was dead. The camera stayed steady, though the time-lapse movie it made moved so quickly I felt dizzy. Hot and sick. The fox lay still as decay did its work. The dirt stole its fur away, bared its snout to the bone. The crack between its lips became a line that stretched until I could see white, the jagged curve of its teeth. And then there was no more fox, only bone. The room spun around me. I coughed again and again. It felt like my throat was full of dirt.

I went back to the doctor and then back again. He shook his head. He said they needed to do some tests. He said they'd take a tube with a camera at the end and slide it through my right nostril so they could photograph my larynx and my trachea, my lungs and airways. The scope would send out a small stream of saline and suck it back in again. They'd be able to see what was wrong with me under the microscope, floating in that fluid, afterward. There would be blood and spit. There would be danger: at the least a low-grade fever, at most one lung collapsed from surrounding air. He motioned my mother out into the hallway then shut the door between them and me. I sat on the examining table, coughing, kicking my legs against its side and listening to the thin white paper rustle in protest.

In the car on the way home, my mother asked me, "Is this about her leaving?"

I answered with silence.

She asked again. "Is this about your teacher?"

I didn't answer. I didn't cough.

14

I DON'T KNOW WHAT HAPPENED, EXACTLY, BETWEEN ME AND my fifth-grade teacher.

I know enough to say this: she never touched me in the ways my mother warned me about, in the places where my arms could cross into an *X*. Sometimes she walked up and down the aisles of desks while she lectured about the water cycle, aqueducts, the human body's resistance to breathing water. Sometimes she paused and then stopped and then stood behind me. I felt her hand on my back, moving in circles. There were her hands, once her lips on my cheek. There's the fact that after my mother said that I couldn't go to her house over Christmas break, my teacher instead extended the offer to Louisa. Louisa accepted, and her mother agreed.

I know that I wasn't molested. I know lines were crossed, but I don't know what those lines were. I don't know how to describe what did happen, or rather the feeling of it: Discomfort. Disquiet. Alarm. I do know that this thing I don't remember, that I didn't and don't understand, came to dominate much of the conversation with doctors about the things that happened as my body stopped being a child and became an adult, which taught me to keep what I felt and experienced as my own secrets.

I wonder: Did I start coughing because my teacher left, or because Louisa was the one who told me, the one who knew first?

I wonder: Was I actually faking the cough that kept me out of school for two weeks? I want to know. I want to remember. But I don't know what I want to remember: that I was faking it, which means that I did have control over my body even if I didn't have control over my emotions, or that I wasn't faking it, which means that I didn't have control over my body or my emotions?

15

When I think about my fifth-grade year, I remember covering a plastic snowflake with glue and glitter to make a Christmas ornament. I remember that the glitter stayed on my fingertips for a week, and how I hung the star so far back in the tree that no light could come from it. Years later, I snapped the snowflake in half. I said it was an accident. I lied.

I remember how many breaths my teacher said I'd take every day. I remember trying to count my breaths. I thought that I could count them all for her. I thought that would bring her back.

I remember the fox, its nest of snow and leaves, and the flesh leaving it for bone. The hook of its jawline, the eye and its pupil that decayed and left behind a socket, a hole. I wanted to run the film backward. I wanted to see time sewing the skin back over the bones. I wanted to see the bite that sliced the fox's jugular disappear. I wanted to believe in a miracle, even if I knew it was impossible. I wanted to see its throat whole, its paws repadded and ready to step with the pack, over and away from the snow.

16

ONE MORNING AND WITHOUT WARNING, BROTHER BENJAMIN took all the boys into the Parish Hall basement and told them that sometimes they'd go to sleep and wake up wet. Mrs. Mallard took the girls into a room in the library none of us knew about, like a secret passage in a mystery movie. She opened a door that looked like part of the wall and made us sit in even rows. The room smelled like a doctor's office: antiseptic, medicated cotton balls, and wooden-sticked swabs. She showed us a video of what was inside of our bodies, pink and red and purple tubes twisting up and around one another like the climbing bars on the playground. Sometimes, she and the video told us, these organs worked together to make a baby. Most of the time, there was no baby, and so these organs made us bleed instead.

I sat on the floor and looked at the blinking red light that appeared on the VCR every time Mrs. Mallard pushed Pause or Rewind. I tried not to correct Mrs. Mallard: We would bleed *excessively*. We would hurt *terribly*. We would panic, thinking we'd have to wear Teenage Softies like Are-You-There-God Margaret.

After the video, we met the boys and Brother Benjamin in the Parish Hall. No one looked at anyone. We were all very relieved when the lights went out, even though it meant a slideshow, which probably meant a quiz. I poked the blue end of my erasable pen into and out of the threads that wove around each other to make my shoelaces. I looked up when I heard the first slide click into place. On the wall, a wash of white-and-blue light turned into a photograph of what Mrs. Mallard said were aborted fetuses, pulled to limbs and lying in wet red stacks in buckets. My stomach rose inside of me and it felt like the time I pushed my body too far up on the swing set. I couldn't look up anymore. I sat and looked at the plastic tube curled around the end of my shoelace. The wall flashed bright and then dark above me.

17

AT FIRST, MY PERIOD SEEMED USEFUL. IT GAVE ME AN EXCUSE to get out of the worst parts of school. If I looked meaningfully at the teacher who blew whistles at us in the gym and said, "I need to go to the bathroom," I would be allowed to go to the bathroom, where I could discreetly draw pictures of cats on the stall door instead of doing jumping jacks.

By my third period, things had changed. Irrevocably. My periods had become so painful that I could no longer focus on drawing cats, discreetly or indiscreetly. My periods soon also became so frequent that the gym teacher questioned my meaningful looks. My Catholic school took both lying and the female reproductive system very seriously, and since the problems with my female reproductive system were so serious that they seemed like lies, I had to see a physician to receive a doctor's note.

The doctor's note confirmed that approximately everything was beginning to go wrong with my female reproductive system. I was diagnosed with dysmenorrhea. My dictionary later classified this as a noun that related to medicine and meant, simply, "painful menstruation," which didn't seem very helpful or clear. It also didn't seem to explain why every time I started my period, I also started to faint and vomit, sometimes at the same time.

"But she's so young. Why is this happening," my mother asked the doctor, "and can you fix it?"

The doctor made a very small noise with his mouth, something like a *phhht*. Were I older, he said, he'd suspect endometriosis, but I was too young for that. He wrote a prescription for naproxen sodium. It didn't stop the cramping, but it dulled the intensity enough for me to go to school, to learn the difference between phyla and kingdoms, between water vapor and mist, between venial and mortal sins, between a made-up story called fiction and a made-up story called a lie.

18

HERE IS WHAT I LEARNED ABOUT ENDOMETRIOSIS AT THE library.

In 1860, the Austrian pathologist Baron Carl von Rokitansky classified a series of anomalies he found in dead female bodies. According to Ronald E. Batt's *A History of Endometriosis*, these anomalies related to "an *excess* of müllerian tissues associated with a normally developed uterus and ovary situated in the interior of a female corpse." In other words, Rokitansky looked inside of dead female bodies and discovered that endometrial tissue, meant to grow only on the inside of the uterus, can grow outside of the uterus. There, it does the same things it does in the uterus. It swells. It sheds. It bleeds.

This is, needless to say, problematic.

When endometrial tissue swells and sheds and bleeds inside of the uterus, the blood and tissue exits through the vagina. When endometrial tissue is outside of the uterus, there's no way for the blood and tissue to exit the body. It hangs around in the female's abdomen, where it makes cysts, irritates tissue, and turns that irritated tissue into adhesions. Those adhesions can, in turn, bind the abdominal organs together and to the pelvic wall.

Batt writes that the current definition of endometriosis—"the microscopic identification of *excess* endometrial glands and stroma located in ectopic locations"—comes directly from Rokitansky's work. In the 154 years since, no one has been able to answer two other questions about endometriosis: *Why* does it happen, and *how* does it happen?

This means that no one has been able to answer a third question: How can we *stop* it from happening?

19

AFTER MY PERIOD SURPRISED ME AND MY FAMILY, MY MOTHER
told me that every day on the way home from elementary school, I
was allowed to ask her one question about anything. She promised
that she would answer it honestly, no matter what. The latter was a
gift that sometimes carried along with it a bonus of utter and abject
embarrassment. By "a question about anything," my mother meant
to imply "a question about what is happening to and inside of your
body and what will happen to and inside of your body in the future."

Most of the questions related to something that Samantha Lee
had whispered into a cluster of ponytailed girls with their heads
bowed on the playground: for example, *Is it true that you can't bathe
when you're on your period?* and *Is it true that if any kind of discharge
comes out down there it can be classified as having a period?* and *What
is discharge and why is it down there?* My mother would close her eyes
briefly, shake her head, and sigh. "Someone needs to call that girl's
mother," she'd say.

When it came to sex, my questions were not particularly well-
formed and generally boiled down to one query: Okay, but what is
the big deal about sex anyway? While we hadn't really learned exactly what it was in school, we'd been told that it was something
that should only be done inside of the confines of a marriage that
took place on consecrated ground sanctified and sanctioned by the
Roman Catholic Church. If we had sex, whatever that was, before we
had entered into the Sacrament of Holy Matrimony on consecrated

ground, it was a mortal sin for which we would not be forgiven until we had confessed and atoned for said sin through the holy Sacrament of Reconciliation.

My mother agreed with the Roman Catholic Church, of course, but she offered an alternative explanation for why sex should only happen inside of a marriage. "Sex can be good," my mother said. "I mean, very good. Eventually." I closed my eyes briefly and sighed, regretting that I had asked the question. "But that takes time. It takes a lot of practice. It's not good the first time. It hurts. It's awkward and it feels like a very animal thing." She turned her head toward me and glanced over the frames of her giant red sunglasses. "That's why you need to be married to someone you love very much and want to be with for the rest of your life, because it takes practice and patience before you get it right." I nodded and tried to separate this information, which seemed like very healthy, good advice, from the fact that the person who delivered this information was my mother, which I didn't want to think about.

20

MY FATHER LET ME CHECK OUT WHATEVER LIBRARY BOOKS I wanted, within reason and as long as he approved them: no nudity, no sex scenes, no too-adult content. One Saturday, I found Freud's *The Interpretation of Dreams*. When I flipped through the book and saw the word *sexual*, I knew I'd hit the jackpot. In a stealth operation, I hid the book between two books about making puppets, which, besides dreams, the word *sexual*, and the Virgin Mary, was one of my main preoccupations. I became brave enough to read it openly during quiet time in Mrs. Kendricks's class. I smelled her approaching before I saw her: White Shoulders and white Tic Tacs. Mothballs and medicinal mouthwash.

"That's an awfully thick book, Emily," she said, the long, gnarled twig of her pointer finger moving toward me. She flipped up the cover just enough to see the title. "Oh no," she said, not in a that-is-something-dangerous kind of way but in a you-will-not-fool-me-young-lady kind of way. "I don't think so." She locked the book in her desk drawer until the bell rang at three, at which point she returned it to me with a definite reluctance.

"This is not an appropriate book for school," Mrs. Kendricks said, lemon-pith bitter. "Please make sure that it does not come back to school with you in the future." She held the book between two fingers as if it were a snake, which, I'd recently discovered, often appeared in the dreams of women experiencing sexual frustration, whatever that may be.

In the car, I held the book in my lap, confessing what had happened to my mother. She glanced at the cover and rolled her eyes.

"That damn library," she said. "That one goes straight back immediately." She looked at me in a kind-of-stern way, but I could tell she was trying not to laugh, which, in dreams, symbolizes an attempt to get rid of unnecessary stiffness.

When Mrs. Kendricks pursed her lips and stopped me, I was reading chapter 3 of *The Interpretation of Dreams*: "The Dream Is the Fulfillment of a Wish." A friend said to Freud: "My wife asked me to tell you that she dreamt yesterday that she was having her menses. You will know what that means." Freud, of course, knew exactly what that meant: his wife was pregnant. That was a terrifying thing for a girl in Catholic school who (1) had actually dreamed that she had started her menses and (2) was already terrified by the idea of the Immaculate Conception.

In other words, Mrs. Kendricks was probably right to take the book away.

21

MY MOTHER DIDN'T TEACH ME HOW TO USE A TAMPON, though it had nothing to do with the rumor I'd heard that if you used a tampon, you were no longer a virgin. "That's absolutely ridiculous," my mother said. "You just don't need to worry about those yet," she said. But in the summer between my sixth- and seventh-grade years, I did indeed need to worry about them. I went to the beach for a four-day trip with my friend Mary, who sang a beautiful, woodwind-toned alto next to my creaking soprano in choir, and her mother. Before we left, I'd counted and recounted the circled dates in my homework planner, checking and rechecking until I was absolutely sure that I wouldn't—or, at least, shouldn't—start my period until I was back home, where I wouldn't have to wear a bathing suit or swim and become shark bait. And then there I was, in the bathroom of a two-bedroom condominium five hours from home, staring with awestruck disbelief at the blood crimsoning its way through my underwear. I'd counted the circles so many times. It'd only been two weeks since my last period.

Then I started to do what I did every time I started my period: I cried. I cramped. I threw up and passed out and threw up again. I bled and bled.

I was completely unprepared and without Kotex, and so the humiliating choice wasn't even a choice. I had to ask my friend's mother for a pad. I stood up and, through the dizzy stars that swirled and swarmed, I opened the door and called her name. When my vision went gray, I thought better of standing and instead sat in the crack that the door made until she appeared, dim and starry, just outside of the bathroom.

"What in the world," she said.

"I started and I don't have Kotex," I said, and I heard her make a noise that sounded like a bird flapping in frustration after finding a windowpane where it should've found sky.

"Oh for Christ's sake," she said, and I agreed but I was also crying, I was saying, "I'm sorry, I'm sorry," and she was asking, "Didn't you *know*?" and I was crying and dizzy and saying, "I'm sorry, I'm sorry." She calmed down and shushed, so I returned the favor. She disappeared. I held my breath to keep from crying. A few minutes later, her hand reached into the bathroom, a long, thin, unrecognizable rectangle inside of it.

"Here," she said, dropping the object into my hand.

She had given me a tampon.

Specifically, she had given me a super-plus absorbency tampon.

It was nearly the size of my hand. I stammer-asked, "But how do I—I've never used one of these?" In the small beam of light cracking through the doorframe, I saw her shake her head. She told me not to be scared and dropped a folded rectangle of paper into my hand. She told me to follow the instructions. It was easy, she said, just super easy.

I unfolded the rectangle to see a Halloween horror version of my mother's doctor's pamphlets.

I looked at the written instructions. They looked back at me.

I couldn't see them as anything but a series of letters blurred into one gray square. "I don't think I can do this," I said.

"Just stick it up there. You'll figure it out when you try," she said. I heard her bedroom door close at the other end of the hallway. She was gone. I sat on the bathroom floor and felt how cool it was and considered, briefly, just sleeping in the bathtub that night.

I stood up slowly, carefully, inch of my body by inch of my body. Stars shot and sparkled over the tile so I counted the seconds—*one Mississippi, two Mississippi*—to have something else to think about. I studied the diagram again, a fun house map of indefinable, inexplicable circles and squiggling lines. I did what the diagram told me to do: I bent my knees. I crouched. I leaned slightly over my stomach. I just stuck it in there.

And then I woke up on the floor, the tampon on the tile, unphased and half-inside of its applicator.

I wasn't sure if the five-second rule applied to tampons, and I was pretty sure that more than five seconds had already passed, anyway. So I did what my own mother taught me to do when, at Sunday mass or my grandmother's house or the grocery store, my period attacked me unawares. I unrolled a long swath of toilet paper and sort-of-folded it into something that looked like a pad. I put the wad of tissue in my panties, said a Hail Mary, then got very carefully and gingerly into the bed.

The morning after I failed to figure out how to use a tampon, I went to the condo's guest shop to buy a package of Kotex. By the time I got back, I realized I wasn't the only one who'd be getting sick in the bathroom that day: Mary's stomach was in the process of rejecting the boil-and-peel shrimp we ate the night before. I felt so relieved and happy that I knew it was a sin, so I closed my eyes and said the Act of Contrition. *O my God, I am heartily sorry for having offended Thee, and I detest all my sins because I dread the loss of heaven and the pains of hell.*

My friend's mother went to the beach while my friend and I spent the day indoors, singing Andrew Lloyd Webber duets as loudly as we could. Because her stomachache had given me a reason for staying home that didn't involve talking to anyone about my period, I let her be Christine while I played the Phantom. I was getting pretty good at it. I was getting pretty good at acting surly and tortured and using my sweaters or T-shirts as a cape. Sometimes I squinted an eye to indicate that something tragic had happened. Sometimes I covered half of my face with my hand.

22

ON THE LAST DAY OF MY BEACH TRIP WITH MARY, I TRIED to use a tampon again. I felt like I owed that to her. She'd been patient and kindly asked very few questions, even after she stopped throwing up shrimp and I still didn't want to get in the pool. I locked the bathroom door. I bent my knees and crouched and when I woke up on the floor, I could tell that I hadn't been unconscious as long this time. This felt like a good sign. My down-there felt strange and bulky and uncomfortable, like part of the tampon was still sticking out. I checked again to see if my down-there matched the down-there in the diagram. It was impossible to tell.

I put on my bathing suit with an attached skirt, just in case—I didn't know much about tampons, but I'd learned from commercials that they're not supposed to be visible, especially when you're swimming, playing beach volleyball, or wearing very tight pants. I walked down the steps of the indoor pool, eyes closed, Hail Marying with every move. I made it to the tile marking the shallow end's three-foot depth before I knew: I had definitely, totally, absolutely not inserted the tampon correctly. By the time I pushed open the door to the ladies' restroom with a desperate, dangerous speed, the tampon had expanded in exactly the same terrifying way that those toy sea creatures in capsules expand from the size of a pill to the size of your palm when left in a bowl of water.

I sat on the toilet and braced myself, just in case I passed out. I pulled the string. I blacked out for only a few starry seconds, which felt like a miracle. Thanking Mary for sort of answering all the Hails I sent her way, I threw the tampon into the trash can, where it landed with a terrifying yet satisfying *thunk*.

For the rest of that last day at the beach, I sat on the side of the pool with my feet in the water, like my grandmother did when she'd just gotten her hair done at JCPenney. I read a Baby-Sitters Club Super Special about their own group trip to the beach, where they felt confident in their swimsuits and ate ice cream and never menstruated or even peed. I went to the hotel gift shop again. I bought a cowrie shell with googly eyes and pipe-cleaner arms that held a tiny guitar. I bought an anklet made of white and pink seashell shards. It scratched my skin to scabs but I wore it anyway. I wanted to make a point. I wanted to pretend that all of this—the staying inside and the sideline sitting—was my choice and my choice entirely. I wanted everyone to think that I was having a good time, such a very good time that I wanted to buy a souvenir to remind me of it.

THE TIGER AND THE CAGE

23

THE FIRST TIME I PASSED OUT, I STOOD IN THE BATHROOM and in the gray light and in my mother's Victoria's Secret nightshirt, looking at myself in the mirror. Then I was no longer in the mirror. When I returned to my body, I discovered that it and I had somehow ended up on the bathroom floor. I was afraid of what my body had done to the me inside of it. I was also afraid that no one would believe what my body had done. I didn't tell anyone.

The second time: my father and I were at the vet with Morgan, my tremendously, handsomely angry cat, for a checkup. I waited in the waiting room while my father paid the bill. Morgan hissed, growled, and spat through his sedation. The room dissolved. I knew that in seconds, I could find myself in my body on the floor next to Morgan and his high, howling complaints. I told my father I'd meet him outside. Then I walked in my body through what looked like clouds. The weather was clear. My body and I made it to the car, somehow, and I sort-of-slumped against the passenger door until I heard footsteps and growling, the click of car doors coming unlocked. I was safe. My secret wasn't.

I told my father that I'd just gotten a little dizzy. That's all. I tried to smile. I didn't want him to worry. "Okay," he said in way a that indicated that he was indeed worried but didn't want to worry me in return. All the way home, he drove quickly and then slowly and then quickly again, and I caught him watching as I slid down a little in the passenger seat. I did not want him to be afraid. I did not want me to be afraid. I tried to position myself in the seat in such a way as to imply I was fine. In the back seat, Morgan hissed at his carrier's door, at the window, at the road and the trees and the sky moving like a movie beyond him.

24

I FAINTED FIVE MORE TIMES BEFORE I TOLD MY MOTHER OR a doctor. I'd learned enough about doctors to know that sometimes it was better to keep my body's secrets. But I was frightened of living inside of a body that wouldn't stop, that fell on the floor and left me behind until it decided to wake me, opening its eyes to the bathroom cabinet, to a gleaming white stretch of tile. I told my mother and then a pediatrician what kept happening.

They did not believe me, exactly.

They believed me inexactly—that I felt dizzy, that I saw stars, that I got a little woozy if I stood up too fast—but they didn't believe me *exactly*. This was, I told myself, my own fault. I'd kept quiet for so long that I didn't know how to describe what my body had done or what it had failed to do. And I couldn't blame them, not really, anyway: it had barely been a year, if that, since I had coughed and coughed.

Here is how my mother began to believe me and exactly: One afternoon, I started up the stairs when I felt it. The slow dissolve of what I knew as myself, of who or what or where I was, in so much starry space. I thudded down and against the wall.

About the scene that followed, I don't remember much in terms of details. I just remember my anger, the seething red distance between preteen daughters and their mothers over which words rarely survive and are never fully understood. She thought I might be faking it. She wanted me to tell her, right then and there, if I was faking it. And if I was faking it, then I'd better stop, right then and there. My pediatrician suspected that I was faking it, she said. They both remembered my cough.

"It's not like that," I told my mother, crying and snotting into my shirtsleeve. "I'm not faking. I'm not faking. I swear to God." Soon, I'd fainted for the eighth and ninth times. Soon, my periods got so bad that I'd sometimes pass out five or six times in one morning. Soon, my parents had to hold up my body so that if I passed out while vomiting I wouldn't choke. It was clear to me and to my parents that I wasn't faking. Still, none of the doctors believed me, exactly.

My mother told me that she understood, that the very same things had happened to her. She sometimes bled like a stuck pig, she said, and spent nights doubled over in a rocking chair moving her body backward and forward through pain, praying that God would just make it stop or at least not make her throw up. She'd passed out when she was my age, too, though her own mother had told her that it was her own damn fault for not sitting down and putting her head between her legs when she started to feel dizzy.

"You know when you're about to pass out," her mother had said, "so there's no reason for you to hit the floor."

She was trying to make me feel less alone, trying to make me realize that other people's bodies did the same things that my body did and that her body just so happened to be one of those bodies. I must have recognized that, somewhere and somehow, even then. Or else I want to think that I must have recognized that, somewhere and somehow, even then. That I wanted to nod and thank her for telling me and tell her that I didn't feel so alone.

That, however, is not the real story.

The real story is that every time she told me that she understood, that her body had also done yet another of the things that my body did to me, I felt them: all of the angers, flaring and spreading throughout my rib cage. Because that's how it happens, sometimes. It's easiest to feel and to say the worst things about the people who love you the most. I told my diary that it drove me crazy, that we weren't the same person and I wished she would recognize that, wished she would let me have at least something of my own, even if it were terrible.

My mother, of course, found the journal and read it. "You were so hateful," she said as she drove me home from school that afternoon, each word a short little bullet. "I don't understand how you can be so hateful. I was just trying to help you. I guess you don't want me to do that anymore." I heard the hurt in her voice.

I confess: part of me hurt, and terribly, to think that I had hurt her.

I confess: part of me felt glad. It felt good, to have something to be angry about. It felt good to be angry about something that wasn't my body, my self.

25

My mother, of course, never for a second stopped trying to help me.

After I'd passed out for the ninth and tenth times, my mother took me to see the pediatrician. He pressed his stethoscope against my chest. He shook his head and clicked his tongue and said he couldn't see a reason for my so-called fainting spells, except that my blood pressure was extremely low. There was nothing to do except make sure I sat down and put my head between my legs when I felt dizzy. He referred me to a neurologist who managed to fit me in to his schedule two months later.

The neurologist wanted to find out if the electrical impulses in my brain acted properly even if they and I hadn't had enough sleep. He scheduled an electroencephalogram for the afternoon of my first day of seventh grade. At the appointment, his nurse parted my thick and ruthless hair down to the scalp, sticking electrodes to the skin with a glue that took weeks to wash out. She told me to lay down on a table as if it were a bed and get comfortable. The table was nothing like a bed. I was not comfortable.

But the test told them nothing, except that everything seemed to happen the way it was supposed to happen in my brain. "There's nothing I can do for her," the neurologist told my mother. He suggested that I see a cardiologist. He suggested that she might want to look for a doctor who treated different aspects of the brain, if she knew what he meant. He gave her a knowing look.

The cardiologist suspected mitral valve prolapse, a syndrome in which the valve between the upper and lower chambers of the heart is a little too thick, a little too fat, which keeps it from closing correctly. As a result, blood can sometimes slip back into the left atrium. We'd know for sure, he said, only if one of his machines caught the sound that thick valves sometimes make, which he called a click. In other words, he could give me a diagnosis if and only if my valve malfunctioned while he was listening.

"But what if it doesn't click when you're listening?" my mother asked.

"Oh, that's very possible," the cardiologist said. "Probable, even. I'd be willing to say she has it, based on her symptoms, but if I don't hear it, I can't confirm it."

My mother and the cardiologist and I watched my heart pulse and push on a monitor, a series of gray spots that, according to the cardiologist, did what they were supposed to do, just fine. He sent me home with a halter monitor. It looked like a dangerous version of a Walkman, headphones replaced with adhesive pads that sucked red circles out of my skin. I wore it for forty-eight uncomfortable hours, during which my valve did what it was supposed to do, just fine.

"He can't make a definite diagnosis," the cardiologist's nurse told my mother, "but wants her to try beta-blockers, just in case." Since my blood pressure was already dangerously low, the beta-blockers could make me faint, constantly. "Just call the nurse and tell her if that happens and we'll figure something out," the cardiologist said.

I tried the beta-blockers. They lowered my blood pressure. They made me faint. Constantly. I spent most of my time sitting down with my head between my legs. Then I had trouble sitting up in the first place. My mother called the nurse and told her what had happened.

"Oh," the nurse said. "I see." She suggested that I see a different kind of doctor. She suggested that I look at Children's Hospital, where there were excellent child psychologists.

26

My Catholic school's parish hall. I was standing by table six, the one manned by Laura's mother, who reportedly tried to pay the Pope to annul her marriage to a man who didn't love her because he loved men. I was standing there mostly because of the story, which was so scandalous I couldn't avoid an obsession with it. I picked up snow globes, turning them over and watching snow gather in glittered clouds then fall, filling the branches of the plastic trees, the rim of the snowman's miniature top hat.

It was the week before Christmas break and the entire seventh grade walked through the parish hall's auditorium, where later we'd gather to sing carols for our parents and godparents and whoever else felt obligated to come and sit and wish they could sleep through our shrill off-notes. Someone took out the rows of folding chairs and replaced them with rows of tables covered in cotton batting and glitter-painted pine cones. Each table was numbered and stacked with presents we were supposed to buy for others, not for ourselves. "Greed is a sin," Father preached in his Advent homilies, "and generosity the greatest of virtues. Remember the loaves and the fishes."

I couldn't stop looking at the snow globe and at the snow inside it, which at my hand's command rose from the bottom then flew to the top, where it floated down again, which could've been, for all I'd seen of it, what real snow did. I picked out a picture frame for my mother, who stood at the front table with the cashbox, and tried to secret it under my arm. I considered a shaving set for my father, with a fat brush meant not for blush but to lather and spread shaving cream.

I stared into the snow globe, at the snowman and the carrot he wore for a nose, at the tiny flecks of something that looked, I guessed, enough like snow. I wondered if I was allowed to be selfish if I'd already been generous. And then I felt it: that crushing crash somewhere in my abdomen, the pain I'd described to the doctor, when he gave me a list of adjectives to choose from, as stabbing. My body broke out in chills and then in fever and then I panicked. I knew what came next. The gray and the stars and their gathering, and then the moment when I was not myself anymore, when I became the gray and the stars and their gathering, when my body folded over. And before I could put down the snow globe, I felt it. Blood. Too warm and too familiar and already too far down my legs.

The parish hall grayed. Someone shook the room and I shook inside of it. I didn't have much time. I walked through the falling dark in the direction of what I thought was the other side of the room, where I knew my mother stood with the other mothers, counting money and stacking it carefully in matched stacks in a money box. I didn't know where my hands or eyes or legs were and despite all our arguments, despite all the times I'd stomped upstairs and slammed my door and written viciously in my journal, the only story I could tell myself was a single word: *mother, mother, mother.*

I watched her look up and see me. I watched her face change into the face she made when she took one look at me and knew what was coming. Then she was beside me and her arm was on my arm, and I tried to say *I'm okay*, I tried not to cry, I tried to say (but quietly, quietly, just for her), *I started again.*

We moved fast through the dark. We stood in the bathroom. I stood in the stall and then I was lying down. I was throwing up. My mother kneeled in the stall with me, pulling back my hair and saying, "It's okay baby, it's okay." I kept throwing up and trying to think, trying to think-pray, trying to think-pray, *Oh God please let no one see me.* The stall turned black and I wasn't throwing up anymore, just making the motions and sounds. Then I was sitting on the toilet. My skirt sat flipped up over my lap and my shorts and panties lay red on the floor. My thighs were red. The paper towels my mother used to wipe off my legs were red.

"It's okay, baby," she said, then she held out my panties and shorts, lifting my legs and putting them through the leg holes then pulling them up to my torso.

"They're wet," I said, and she said, "I know, Peanut, but we've got to get you home." She handed me a wad of paper towels to stick in my panties, so I stuck them in my panties. We walked out of the stall and I stood and watched my mother as she rolled out and rolled out and rolled out more towels, teeth clenched so tightly her jaw-line looked white. She'd seen this before, of course, because she'd experienced this before—though, she would later tell me, "What I went through is nowhere near what you went through." And even in the half-light of my consciousness, even with pain ringing red in my body, I knew, standing there in the bathroom, why she'd told me so many times that our experiences were similar. Because I wouldn't be standing alone. Because she'd stood where I was standing. Because she understood.

In the car, I sat on the stack of towels. I closed my eyes. I listened to our car's hazard lights do what they do, clicking on, clicking off. I thought about the snow globe. I thought about all of that winter, how I wanted to keep it in my hands. I thought of sin and selfishness. "God finds a way to punish your sins," Father said, "whether you know them as sins or not. God knows."

27

MY MOTHER CAN'T REMEMBER: SHE EITHER SAW A REPORT about the fourth doctor on the news or read an article about him in a magazine. Either way, she just had a feeling that Dr. Four might, finally, be the one to give me a way to solve the equation of my body and stop it from falling, unconscious, on the floor. Dr. Four had discovered that along with their fatter, flubbing heart valves, mitral valve prolapse patients all seemed to carry the same set of symptoms: fainting, fatigue, palpitations, dizziness, numbness. He opened an umbrella term over these symptoms: *dysautonomia*.

Here is what that term means: if it is working correctly, the part of the peripheral nervous system called the autonomic nervous system sends messages that make the human body move and function like it should. These messages travel over the nerves connecting the brain to its body. They tell the heart how fast it should be beating. They tell the stomach how quickly it should digest food, the lungs how quickly they should inhale and exhale. They tell the genitals if it's time to pee or to have sex. If the human body is in danger, the autonomic nervous system kicks into high gear, urging the body to fight or take flight.

Sometimes, Dr. Four had discovered, the autonomic nervous system fails. It tells the heart to pump too fast. The lungs to breathe too quickly. It drops blood pressure. Blurs vision. Dries the mouth. Informs the genitals that even though they are in a romantic situation, they have no business having sex. It can send so many mixed messages that the body won't know what to do or how to do it. Like an overloaded switchboard, the body shorts out.

Dr. Four was too busy to offer me an actual appointment as an actual patient. He could, his receptionist told my mother, offer me an appointment with his nurse—and, more importantly, with the diagnostic machines his nurse operated. By then, I passed out so often that we were desperate. "Anything," my mother said into the phone. "Anything."

At my appointment, Dr. Four's nurse worked fast, as if her goal was actually to move me through and out of the office as quickly as possible—which was, of course, her actual goal. She wrapped a blood pressure cuff around my arm, pulling it taut before securing it with Velcro. She hooked me to a machine that translated the messages sent by my nerves into waves and crests and numbers. Then she handed me a pink balloon and told me to blow it up.

I looked at the balloon. I looked at her. "Are you serious?" I tried to see her eyes, which, it seemed, hadn't actually looked at Actual Me, just the graphs and numbers and charts related to Inside Me. She *huh*ed to indicate confusion then *yes*ed to indicate annoyance. She held the balloon a little closer to me and shook it, as if I were a dog who hadn't quite seen its owner's stick. I took the balloon and blew it up until I couldn't see her nose or eyes, just her eyebrows, which seemed at first crestfallen but then lifted in a pleased kind of way. She let out a hopeful *oh*. I tried to look at the machines, but they were as unhelpful as she was, and besides, I was feeling dizzy.

"Are you feeling dizzy?" The nurse kept her eyes on those waves and crests and I realized that's what they were telling her, that the language they shared was the one with which my body told itself to faint. It felt strange, to be on the outside of a conversation in which my body explained itself, finally.

I moved the balloon away from my mouth. "I am feeling very dizzy," I said. "Can I please stop now?"

28

DR. FOUR WAS IMPORTANT BECAUSE HE WAS ONE OF THE FEW doctors who could perform a tilt table test, the primary method for diagnosing dysautonomia.

Here is how it works: A person lays down on this table that looks like the table Dr. Frankenstein used. A nurse straps the person onto the table, then hooks them up to machines that measure heart rate and blood pressure. Then the table moves upward at an angle while the nurse watches the machines. If the patient's autonomic nervous system works correctly, it tells her body to adjust to this change in position. It tells her heart to speed up. It tells the blood vessels in her legs to shrink so that her blood moves normally throughout the body as a whole. As a result, the patient won't faint.

If, however, a person's autonomic nervous system isn't sending the right kind of messages, their body will become dizzy. The body will see stars. The body will pass out.

I remember laying down flat on the table. I remember being hooked up to machines. I remember the nurse's hand, which patted and then kept its place on my arm as she explained that she was about to turn on the table, that I'd travel upward until my body was sort-of-standing, that I might feel a little dizzy and I should tell her if I did. I nodded and closed my eyes, preparing to monitor my symptoms.

She turned on the table. I remember that: the quickening buzz of electricity, the expectation, if not the feeling, of motion. I remember a swarm of tiny bright lights buzzing into my field of vision. I remember the words swarming in my mind and my mouth, which opened to let them out: *I have become dizzy.* I don't remember anything else.

When my mother tells the story, she says the table had just started to tilt my body upward when the machines sounded their alarms. The nurse's eyes popped open, widened, alert, and I imagine in this moment she felt a kind of recognition that maybe I was someone to pay attention to after all. My mother tells me that the nurse said, "Whoa-oh," just like that, like two separate words, the *whoa* deep and slow and the *oh* pitched high and fast. She shut off the table. After a few minutes of stillness, my body calmed down. I returned to myself.

"I've never had anyone respond so quickly," the nurse told my mother. "I want to see something," she said. "Would you mind holding her knees?"

I remember, dimly, realizing what she meant: she wanted to see exactly how far—or rather, how *not* far—the table had to tilt before I passed out completely. I remember, dimly, realizing that even though it was my body that she wanted to study, she didn't ask my permission.

I started to cry. I told myself to stop. I told myself: *They're going to think you're dramatic. They're going to think you're faking. They're going to think you're a faker, so suck it up.* And so I swallowed and closed my eyes and bit the insides of my cheeks to keep myself from crying. The nurse checked the machines, checked the straps, checked their buckles. My mother held on to my knees in case they buckled.

The table went up. I went out.

29

THIS IS THE PART WHERE MY OWN STORY IS NO LONGER MY own because my body is no longer my own.

There I am, in my body, lying on the bathroom floor.

There I am, sweating and fevered and wishing I could feel the tile, which I remembered should be cool.

There I am, bleeding through two overnight Kotex, passing blood clots half the size of my own hand and terrified because I am too young to know that an internal organ hasn't fallen out.

There I am, without the language to ask for help. There I am fainting and there are my parents, there is my father holding the bulk of my body up and over the toilet, there is my mother. She's wiping my face with a wet washcloth. She's holding my head up and back by the ponytail to keep me from aspirating, there I am fainting and vomiting at the same time, there I am under my parents' hands, moving the bulk of my body from floor to toilet, there I am shitting uncontrollably while throwing up into the trash can someone put on the floor below me. There I am, the person I cannot remember as a person, the person detached from her being, from her body, who no longer lived inside of a story she could understand.

30

I ALWAYS HAVE STRANGE AND PERSISTENT RECURRING dreams.

For example: I fall asleep in a dream and wake up in the dream. I look at my bedroom window. I am not alone in looking at my bedroom window. Something is out there, glow-eyed and glaring, some huge, hungry tiger waiting to strike.

For example: I'm sitting in the passenger seat of my mother's car, watching her steer. I fall asleep inside of the dream and wake up inside of the dream, in the passenger seat of my mother's car. I realize I'm alone. I realize my mother is no longer steering the car. I realize that I have no idea how to drive.

For example: I'm standing on the balcony of the condominium where my family stayed at the beach. I'm watching the ocean. I'm watching its waves, gathering and cresting and reaching out over the shore. I'm watching its waves gather and crest and reach and then I know: the wave is coming for me.

Even in the dream, there is nothing I can do.

31

THE THING I REMEMBER MOST ABOUT DR. FOUR'S OFFICE wasn't the blood pressure cuffs or balloons. It wasn't the tilt table and the buckles, or the machines and the wires they used to help my body tell them what it was doing. It wasn't the fear or the dizziness or the fainting. What I remember most was the excitement that hummed electric through the air, the atmosphere of pure jubilation. That day, the nurses and doctors and machines had made a discovery that could change the way that the medical community thought about dysautonomia. They thought their discovery could prove, once and for all, that dysautonomia was a real and actual thing.

This discovery had nothing to do with me or my body or the fact that I'd passed out faster than any patient they'd seen. In fact, while the severity of my symptoms did give me a definite diagnosis, it didn't give me much else—including an appointment with Dr. Four himself. He was still too busy. He was probably going to be even busier, the nurses surmised, because of the miracle that had happened right there, in that very lab, on that very tilt table, recorded by those very machines.

The miracle was this: they had discovered and diagnosed a case of dysautonomia in a boy.

I was diagnosed with dysautonomia when I was twelve. Even after my tilt table test, my mother and I rarely told doctors about it. We tried, at first, but the doctors pushed their lips together and closed their eyes in a lingering way and nodded, very gently, as if they'd just understood something important. "I see," the doctors would say, and then they'd offer referrals to Children's Hospital, where there were many good doctors who could help me with what was wrong inside of my head.

They were not referring to my nervous system.

Dr. Four's nurse tried to explain what happened to my body when I passed out. "Imagine that you are a tiger in a cage," she said, and so I imagined a tiger in a cage. I imagined the exact same tiger who, glow-eyed and glaring, waited at the window of my dreams. "Now imagine that tiger gets spooked and feels threatened," she said, and so I turned the tiger I dreamed from the threat into the threatened. "That's what's happening. Your body is the cage. Your autonomic nervous system is the tiger. You could be just sitting there on the couch, perfectly still, and your autonomic nervous system will act like that, like a tiger who gets scared."

I imagined my body as a cage. I imagined a tiger inside of it. What I couldn't imagine was the connection between them, the cause that made the effect. "How does the tiger get scared?" I asked. "How do I stop that from happening?"

I wanted a definitive answer. I wanted to know how to gain control. Instead, she pursed her lips together. She shifted from left to right. She handed my mother a poorly xeroxed handout with tips for controlling dysautonomia: avoid processed sugar and white flour, eat salt and drink lots of water, keep a card in your wallet to notify paramedics that your blood pressure is naturally bottom-of-the-bottom low. She and the handout told me that there are certain known triggers: moments of extreme emotion, the shift in hormone levels during puberty, before menstruation, during pregnancy.

Neither she nor the handout state the obvious: These triggers are unavoidable. The body cannot be tamed out of change.

My mother thanked her and folded the handout into a square small enough to fit in her purse. We walked to the parking deck and slid into the car. We were startled into sneezing by the bright sun, and nothing was different from the moment we parked except that this strange force in my body now had a name.

32

SEVEN YEARS LATER, I SAT IN MY DORM ROOM IN NEW YORK, in a child's soccer T-shirt and jeans and bowling shoes, the phone to one ear and my finger in another, trying to block out my neighbor's ska music so I could understand what my mother was saying.

Even when I heard the words, I couldn't understand her.

She'd called from the hospital, where my father lay flat in a white bed. That morning, he'd been drinking coffee. And then he slid down, unconscious, in his chair. My mother found my father sitting there, blinking with confusion. "He thought everything was fine," she said. "He didn't even know he'd passed out."

My father had said that he didn't need to go to the hospital. "He's just as stubborn as you are," my mother said. "He just kept saying, 'I'm fine, I'm fine,' and I told him, 'You're not fine, you're almost on the floor and that isn't fine.'" Then he passed out again, and my mother insisted on riding down the street to the fire station so they could take his blood pressure. As they walked in, he started to pass out again. The firemen pulled over a folding chair and Velcroed a cuff to his arm. When they measured his blood pressure, it was alarmingly low. "He finally stopped fighting me," my mother said. "He finally stopped saying he was fine."

I nodded and then remembered I was on the phone and needed to speak. "So how is he now?"

"He's fine," she said. "He's tired but he's tired of being here. He's just like you. He gets cabin fever. He's going to drive me crazy."

I nodded into the phone again, almost in time to the ska music's beat.

After a round of wires and electrodes and computers and blood tests, the doctors had their diagnosis: dysautonomia. Just like me.

After my father's diagnosis, I told doctors I had dysautonomia. I watched their eyebrows rise.

"Diagnosed with a tilt table," I'd say, and their eyes closed in that lingering way.

"My father has it, too," I'd say. Their eyes opened. They nodded, not gently, as if something has just become clear. They wrote the words on my chart.

"Make sure you drink enough water," they'd say, "and stay away from processed foods and starch."

PUTTING THE DAMAGE ON

33

Early in the summer after I turned eleven, before mosquitoes stormed the Alabama air and everything smelled like citronella and sweat, my grandmother took my cousin Jessica and me to Gulf Shores. We bought plastic buckets at Walmart and shoved wet sand into them. I overturned them—slowly, carefully—to make a cul-de-sac of sandcastles that Jessica overturned into ruins, one by one, with quick flicks of her feet. I walked to the edge of the ocean when my skin was sun-pinked and stepped in just past the foam, which was as far as I could let myself step. From far out in the water, Jessica waved at me, laughing. The green reached the tops of her shoulders. She jumped sideways into the waves. Because we were both only children, she was the closest thing I had to a sister. I hated her as much as I loved her.

In the mornings, I had my grandmother to myself, which was how I liked it. We walked on the beach, our footprints beading the hem of the Gulf. Sometimes I stopped to pick up tiny mollusks, iridescent and iris, the walls of their homes still pressed together. I dropped them into a bucket of sand and seawater and took them back to the condo's balcony, where I sat cross-legged and watched them dig themselves deeper, letting out their bubbles of air. We always left the beach before I knew for sure if they'd survived in the buckets I'd tried to turn into the sea.

The day before we left, there was a fight. My cousin Jessica said something. I said something back. What we said didn't matter: I yelled and she yelled back, "*So*," and then it was over. My body went electric and all I could see was heat. I didn't even realize that I was screaming until my grandmother told me to get my ass out on the balcony and cool it down.

"*Fine*," I yelled. The volume of my voice at first frightened me. Then I realized my volume felt satisfying, and so I yelled again. "I would be *happy* to. Happy." I tried as hard as I could to slam the sliding glass door, but it was too heavy. It took me two tries to close it, so I hit it with the palm of my hand for emphasis.

I stood in the night and tried not to notice the moon, how small it was, how bright it was, by the Gulf and away from cities and their lights. I tried not to see how the stars looked reflected in the bay, all shine and shimmer against the slow, subtle waves. I tried not to notice the circles of light pearled around the dock. I could see, if I squinted and pushed my glasses all the way up and against my face, the small dots that were crabbers out to pull up their traps. I started to play the game I usually played when I saw crabbers, where the only rule was to count how many seconds passed between the moment they bent down and the moment they stood up with their buckets of crabs. Then I remembered that I was supposed to be angry, and I felt even angrier because I'd forgotten. I couldn't do anything right, even just staying angry. I started to cry, shrill and slobbering. I wanted Jessica to hear me. I wanted my grandmother and grandfather to hear me. I wanted the upstairs and downstairs and left and right neighbors to hear me. I wanted the crabbers to hear me, and the crabs in their buckets, and the crabs still in the bay, scuttling and spitting bubbles across the sand. I knew how I looked, how I sounded: hysterical in all the worst ways. *This is ridiculous*, part of me said. *You have to stop.* The rest of me answered, *I can't.* And this was the first time I felt it, the way I'd feel at the same time every month for years, as if some force had tipped my body headfirst into a darkness I had no choice but to claim.

When I stopped to drag a breath into and out of my body, I heard a neighbor's door slide shut. I was pleased and encouraged, and so I began to get serious. I cried so hard I sputtered. I choked. I thought about jumping off the balcony and landing splat on the concrete landing underneath. As soon as I thought it, I thought someone should hear me say it. I thought everyone should hear it, so they'd know just how serious this was.

"I should just *jump*," I yelled. "I should just *jump* because no one will miss me."

The door opened.

My grandmother's hand circled my arm. She was not gentle. "That's *enough*, Emily," she hissed as she pulled me inside. She told me to splash cold water on my face. She told me to get in that bedroom, get ready for bed, and get quiet, for Christ's sake. She didn't want to look at me and she did not want to hear a single sob or word. She was that serious.

Later, when my mother told my grandmother that I'd started my period, my grandmother was not surprised. She had two sisters, four daughters, six sisters-in-law. She had seen this before, a darkness branching through the women on both sides of our family tree, one that emerged every month, clockwork-precise. She knew there would be no relief until that clock stopped. "I wondered what was wrong with her," she said. "Dealing with her at the beach made me want a drink. A very, very strong drink."

34

AT THIRTEEN, I SWITCHED SCHOOLS. I MOVED FROM SEVENTH grade at my Catholic school, with its prim uniforms and gilded paintings of a prissy, perfectly coiffed Jesus Christ, to eighth grade at the fine arts school downtown. There were no paintings of Jesus at the fine arts school, but there was another absence that felt nothing less than miraculous: there was no gymnasium, which meant I could go to school without the unspeakable humiliations of gym class.

The art school sat in the corner of a square it shared with the juvenile detention center, the prison, and the bus station with its magical and illegal cigarette machine, all of which I was expressly forbidden to even think about going anywhere near. I had been to the bus station, though I hadn't yet put quarters into the cigarette machine or a cigarette into my mouth. I had older friends. Some of them had cars.

Some of them were boys, and some of them were boys who had boyfriends. I majored in creative writing and I used the word *shit* in a short story that my classmates described as *real* and *gritty*. I heard terms like *blow job* and *deep-throating*. I tried to use *deep-throating* in another story, which my classmates also celebrated as real and gritty except for the fact that I had used *deep-throating* as a synonym for "French kissing," which it apparently definitively was not. I was briefly embarrassed but nonetheless still proud that I had heard and repeated the term, and that here, unlike my old school, there was no Sister Nathaniel and therefore no getting sent to Sister Nathaniel's office.

In eighth grade, when the numbers in my algebra book met up with letters, it felt unfamiliar and unfair. All my art school class-mates seemed as nauseated and dizzy as I was, no matter which art they studied. Knowing that they also suffered in nauseous and dizzy confusion both did and did not make me feel better, in the way that letters did and did not make numbers.

"There's one guiding principle behind mathematics," our teacher said. "Elegance. That's what drives every equation: elegance. Beauty." He was trying to be helpful. We sat in our desks and our ripped jeans and black T-shirts and stared at him, just stared, until he sighed and turned around to write another equation on the board.

That afternoon, I'd struggle with my homework in the gynecol-ogist's waiting room. Linear equations. I showed my work. I got an answer. I checked the back of the book and saw that I was wrong. Again. That was the year that doctors started telling me that if I wanted to have a baby, I'd better do it quick. I'd better do it young. I'd need to finish school, of course. I'd need to get a degree, of course. But I'd need to find a nice young man to settle down with, too—and fast. Then I could have a baby followed quickly by a hysterectomy.

I was thirteen.

35

On July 3, 1980, the United States Conference of Catholic Bishops released a statement forbidding Catholic hospitals from performing procedures or prescribing treatments that render the patient incapable of producing offspring. This includes procedures or treatments performed or prescribed for medical reasons. Though this particular statement relates to tubal ligation, its scope was, for many years, extended to all hysterectomies on women who hadn't experienced menopause. Only in 2019 did the Vatican clarify the circumstances in which a hysterectomy would be acceptable: when and only when doctors know, and with certainty, that no future pregnancy would be viable. Therefore, if doctors do not know and with certainty that a fetus couldn't survive in a uterus, said uterus cannot be removed in a Roman Catholic hospital. The procedure would, in the eyes of the Magisterium of the Roman Catholic Church, be forbidden, and everyone involved in this procedure— from the patient to the doctors and nurses and pharmacists who prescribed pain pills and techs who handed over rolls of gauze— would have been party to an act grievous enough to be considered a mortal sin.

On the day that the United States Conference of Catholic Bishops released their statement, I had been alive for forty-nine days. There were still approximately 2 million oocytes, or immature eggs, inside of my body, which, as far as I know, had not yet begun to experience much in the form of pain.

•

On their website, the Mayo Clinic maintains a list of Diseases and Conditions that can affect the female reproductive system. The primary Disease and Condition affecting my particular reproductive system is endometriosis: the abnormal growth of endometrial tissue outside of the uterus. I also experienced the following Diseases and Conditions: adenomyosis, which means that extra endometrial tissue grew into the muscles of my uterus; a fibroid tumor that grew from the size of a Ping-Pong ball to the size of a lemon to the size of a small grapefruit; frequent urinary tract infections (UTIs), kidney stones, and urinary retention; polycystic ovary syndrome (PCOS); hemorrhagic cysts; hemorrhagic implants of endometrial tissue inside of surgical scars; hemorrhagic growths composed of endometrial tissue in various locations in my abdomen, including on my appendix; appendicitis; oligomenorrhea, which means I sometimes skipped periods; polymenorrhea, which means that I sometimes had multiple periods in a month; menorrhagia, which meant I bled through a U by Kotex® AllNighter® Pad in an hour; menometrorrhagia, which meant I sometimes bled through a U by Kotex® AllNighter® Pad when I wasn't even officially having a period; anemia; and adhesions that glued the organs in my pelvis together and then to my pelvic wall.

36

THE FIRST TIME I SAW A GYNECOLOGIST, HE TOLD ME THAT A lot of strong and successful women walked around with the very same things happening in their bodies every day. Endometriosis wasn't dangerous, he said. It wouldn't kill me, but it might keep me from feeling like a normal teenager. He wrote a prescription for stronger painkillers than the pediatrician had prescribed as well as stronger anti-nausea medicine. He wrote a third prescription but said that he couldn't give it to me yet—not until I took a pregnancy test.

My throat closed in on itself. The room grayed. "Excuse me," I said. It was both a question and a plea. I couldn't say what my mind was thinking, what my post-Catholic-schoolgirl mind could not help but think: *How can this be, since I do not know man?*

"Oh no, no, no." The gynecologist laughed. He and his nurse and my mother assured me that no one actually suspected that I was actually pregnant. "We just legally have to do it," his nurse said. "It's just something with the law."

I listened to their hushed assurances and shook my head, again and again.

37

I WAS ALLOWED TO AUDITION FOR THE FINE ARTS SCHOOL AS long as it was in writing or visual art and not theater. "No way," my mother said when I asked about auditioning for the drama department. "Everyone wants to be an actor or an actress and very, very few people make it." Writing, at least, would prepare me for a better future. Writing was a skill practiced by people who were intelligent and successful, like lawyers. My mother said she was saving me from disappointment, and the truth is that she was right.

If I had any talent as an actress, it was no more than any average-to-below-average theater kid, and any talent that I had would quickly be erased by the front teeth bucking out under my braces, my bad skin, and my bad hair. But there was something about acting that felt right nonetheless, something about standing in that lit space and slipping someone else into one's body, slipping words that someone had polished into eloquence over the tongue and out past the teeth. Even if it was just for the length of a ten-minute skit about a group of girls lost on a beach, it was good to move inside a new set of possibilities, to be someone who wasn't the self you usually had to be.

38

THOUGH ENDOMETRIOSIS HAS BEEN MENTIONED IN MEDICAL texts for 4,000 years, no one can explain exactly what it is or exactly why it exists. There are, of course, theories. Some doctors believe it's genetic, passed down from mothers to their daughters. Others believe it's just something that sometimes happens inside of the female body. At the time of my diagnosis in 1993, I heard the most about a theory developed in the 1920s. This theory, promoted by a doctor named John Sampson, claimed that endometriosis happened when menstrual tissue flowed backward up into the fallopian tubes and, from there, settled like seeds into the fertile soil of a woman's pelvis and grew. He called this process retrograde menstruation. Later, studies revealed that while 90 percent of women experience retrograde menstruation, only 6 to 10 percent of women develop endometriosis. Even so, 100 percent of my doctors have believed that retrograde menstruation is the most likely the cause of endometriosis.

Mercury is in retrograde 24.657 percent of the year; however, according to a Gallup poll, only 28 percent of American women and 23 percent of American men believe in astrology and the idea that Mercury's retrograde motion can plant the seeds of mayhem in the fertile soil of our daily lives.

39

My first week of arts school was also the week I realized that I was going to die. I could not stop thinking about it. Scowling at the *X*s and *Y*s in my Algebra I book, hunched over my typewriter in the creative writing classroom, choking down instant mashed potatoes in the cafeteria: I could not stop thinking about it. I hid in the bathroom, trying to avoid my own face as I passed the mirror. I locked the door to the stall and stood inside of it, thinking the same sentence over and over with emphasis on different words, as if I believed I could make myself believe it: *You* are going to die. You *are* going to die. You are *going* to die. You are going to *die.*

When panic closed my throat, when I felt so dizzy I wondered if I was already dead, I stopped myself and said a Hail Mary. Before I got to her being full of grace, my head felt like spinning again. I knew that even those words were just words. Empty. Nothing. It was like the terrible game I played where I'd say my own name over and over again, out loud—"Emily, Emily, Emily, Emily"—like my mother did when she was calling me in from playing too close to the street. After a while *Emily* didn't sound like my name, like anyone's name. It didn't even sound like a word, just a collection of sounds. I didn't know what an Emily was or how I was one. My head filled with sound the way it did when I was standing beneath the school bell as it started its long call for a fire drill, and the sound was so loud and so long that it wasn't even sound anymore, just the indiscriminate terror of ringing and buzzing and alarm that flushed my face and filled my feet with the need—not desire—to run.

40

AFTER MY FIRST APPOINTMENT WITH THE GYNECOLOGIST, my mother stopped in front of my new school's gray concrete walls. It was built to look like a factory, an art factory, all cinder block and unfinished ceilings that were supposed to indicate an industrious dedication to our studies. It was hideous. My mother handed me the doctor's note I was to hand to the gray-haired receptionist in the office.

I looked at the note.

I didn't leave the car.

I imagined the gray-haired receptionist seeing the doctor's name and thinking the word that now seemed too painful for me to say or think: *gynecologist*. I imagined her saying *oh* and raising one gray eyebrow, one side of her mouth. It occurred to me that everyone would know. Instantly. Everyone would know that a stranger had touched me in that place, that I had peed into a cup, that I had cried in a wet, snotty way while the nurse rubbed zeros into my back. Everyone would know that tucked in my mother's purse was the prescription for birth control pills the doctor had given me once he was sure I was not pregnant. And no one would know why I was prescribed them—they'd all just assume I was a bad girl who did bad things.

"Everyone's going to *know*," I said to my mother, and in my own voice I could hear myself wheeling toward crying. She made the sound in her throat that meant she was annoyed, which she sometimes did not out of anger but as a way to signal that this was a big girl moment and I had to learn not to cry.

"For God's sake, Emily," she said, "it's not like you have to wear them around your neck. No one's going to know. And you're late for class." The conversation was over. I kissed her on the cheek and told her I loved her. I left the car. I gave the doctor's note to the gray-haired woman in the office, who said, "Thank you," and "You're good to go," and did whatever she did with all our doctor's notes. I walked the gray stairs in the gray stairwell to Mr. Harden's Algebra I class, where he'd already covered the board with numbers and letters and all the marks that were supposed to connect them.

A few weeks later, a friend made a Pope hat from the poster board left over from my successful bid to become parliamentarian of the student government association. He decided to rebaptize all the members of the school's creative writing department, and if he liked you, he'd let you choose your own name. Otherwise, he'd baptize you as Percy Lumpkinpuss, a name he first bestowed upon Chad, who sat next to me and was such an asshole that I was madly in love with him. He had read *The Communist Manifesto* six times and he could correctly pronounce and define the word *bourgeoisie*, and even spell it. He had called my first poem of the semester childish and did not appreciate the valentine I handmade from a paper doily just for him. I was happy to see him humiliated.

When my friend put on his Pope hat and offered to rebaptize me, I took it very seriously. I chose a name close enough to *Emily* to make sense—*Emma*, for Emma Thompson, for the moment in *Howards End* when she fell in front of the mirror and unpinned her hat and cried in gulps so perfect that I attempted to imitate her every time I cried. I'd watched the movie so many times that the VHS tape slowed and then snapped completely.

As my friend mumbled in close-enough-to-Latin above me, I kneeled and closed my eyes. I felt something shift within me, gears turning and turning one another. The lock locked. I was an Emma, and I could pretend that I had never been an Emily, passed out on the floor of the gymnasium's bathroom, mocked as Emily Boulder-Butt Bolden, teacher's pet and cat-loving nerd. Emily could stay hidden inside the bathroom forever, saying her name to herself again and again and again.

41

1996. THE SUMMER OF MY TENTH-GRADE YEAR AND MY fourth year at a camp where middle and high school students took college-level courses. We called it nerd camp with great affection and pride. My best friend and I had big plans for the dance. We wore our best dresses, spent half an hour on our makeup: frosted blue eye shadow, three coats of mascara, cat-eyed liquid eyeliner thicker than our mothers would ever allow. And then we ran, giggling and holding our skirts, to the water fountain. We closed our eyes and splashed water on our faces, then rushed back to our room. We stood in front of the mirror together to watch our makeup run, just like the model on the cover of Hole's *Live Through This*. We clouded the air with Aqua Net and tossed our heads a few times, like the heavy metal bands we'd once watched on *Headbangers Ball*. We sang along with Courtney Love, our idol. We asked an unnamed someone to go on. We asked them to take everything. We sang that we wanted them to.

Courtney Love. Tori Amos. Alanis Morissette. Liz Phair. No Doubt–era Gwen Stefani. We spent the summer listening and singing and sometimes screaming along with them. We loved them for their anger, for their bravery, for their strength. But I didn't focus on their strength. I focused on their ability not only to admit that they were broken but to articulate *how* they were broken, and where and when, and who had broken them. I envied their ability to confess. To declare. To admit that sometimes, they had broken themselves.

After we'd danced awkwardly with boys and friends and

ourselves, after we'd showered and slipped into our pajamas, my friend smoked a cigarette out of the window. I continued our conversation from my bed, where I buried my head under the quilt my mother made for me before I was born. I tried to act casual. Cool. To pretend I wasn't panicking inside over someone breaking the rules. She tossed the cigarette butt out of the window. I crawled out of bed to shoot Freesia body spray into the air. When my parents picked me up the next morning, I told them I'd burned popcorn before they even said anything about the smell.

On the long drive home, I put *Boys for Pele* into my Discman and lay down in the back seat. I listened to one song over and over: "Putting the Damage On."

42

SOME NIGHTS, WHEN PAIN SCREAMED SO LOUDLY THAT I HAD to admit its presence, I lay on my couch with the pillows stacked in such a way as to hold up my head, which I turned toward the television. I usually watched The Learning Channel. When the clock ticked past eleven, documentaries about human sexuality and all its ceremonies—attraction, courtship, and flirtation—appeared.

From them I learned that women darken their lips and eyelids and cheeks because their lips and eyelids and cheeks darken in approximately the same way during sexual intercourse. This darkening is caused by the influx of blood flow that accompanies an orgasm, which, the programs informed me, is what happens when sexual intercourse is pleasurable and successful. Therefore, the programs also told me, when a woman uses lipstick and eye makeup and blusher before, say, a third date, it's a way of very subtly and smoothly saying, *This is how I will look should you choose to have sexual intercourse with me, which will be pleasurable and successful, so perhaps we could engage in sexual intercourse after these cocktails and steaks?*

The use of red nail polish, The Learning Channel told me, could also be considered a way of flirting. The color red is associated with a woman's menstrual cycle. This means that if a man looks at a woman's fingernails and sees that they are red, that man will, on a subconscious level, connect the color with menstruation and sexual maturity, though more in an indirect *look at that mature lady* kind of way than a direct *that lady is 100 percent menstruating and I am into that* kind of way.

From the prime-time sitcoms that saturated major network television during the 1990s, I learned even more. I learned that *flirting* is the name for a set of human behaviors that may involve but are not limited to: rapid blinking of eyes, the application of mascara and eyeliner, laughter that sounds very little like actual laughter, and sliding smoothly off a barstool in a way that indicates tremendous physical fitness. I learned that *flirting* is often the kick-starter to both minor tensions and major conflicts. Minor flirting-related tensions were usually solvable within the span of thirty minutes; it might take an entire season or more to resolve major conflicts, which typically ended in a wedding, a baby, and/or cancellation of the show.

43

WHERE ARE YOU ON THE KINSEY SCALE?

It's the question we liked to ask one another, in the hallways of the art high school built to look like a factory, as we ran then sock-slid down the tiled hallway, red as a warning. As a command. *Stop.*

Where are you on the Kinsey Scale? Alfred Kinsey and his team of sexuality researchers developed their scale in the 1940s to describe the way that people's bodies react to other people's bodies. In Kinsey's study, most people described sexuality in terms of absolutes: heterosexual or homosexual, no in-betweens. Kinsey, himself bisexual, thought differently. He saw human sexuality not as two opposing points but as a line on which we slide, depending upon the human bodies that our human bodies meet. In the city library, we poured through Kinsey's reports: *Sexual Behavior in the Human Male, Sexual Behavior in the Human Female. Where are you on the Kinsey Scale?* We whispered to one another. To ourselves.

Quietly we snuck the question out of the library, which we'd mapped in our minds. We knew where to hide to kiss or to cry, where we could stand unseen long enough for half a cigarette, shifting our bodies with the smoke into the wind. *Where are you on the Kinsey Scale?* We snuck into school, tiptoed bent-backed past lit classrooms to the bathroom. We washed the aftertaste of smoke from our fingers. Scoured our mouths with Listerine, with the toothbrushes we used to gag ourselves after lunch.

In that building, everything seemed defined by opposing prepositions: on and off, over and under, above and below. I no longer understood the self I saw in photographs: Long hair. Wide cheeks. New boobs. *Where are you on the Kinsey Scale?* Seven words I kept inside my mouth as I watched my face cave, slimmed by skipped lunches. I sheared my hair into a shape I shared with the boys in algebra class. I wore oxford-cloth shirts and oxblood shoes. I wore a rust-colored sweater vest and grey corduroy pants. I spelled *gray* as *grey* until my teacher's red ink told me I had one more chance and then that was it, I'd see an F.

In algebra, I learned that numbers live on an endless line with zero as its middle. Between each number lives an infinity of numbers. There exists an endless series of ways to move toward and away. I learned that the Greeks defined zero as a paradox: How could nothing be something? How could absence be presence? *Where are you on the Kinsey Scale?* For all my asking, I had no idea how to answer when the question turned toward me. At first I said zero, by which I meant nothing, until I found out that in Kinsey's terms, a zero instead meant absolute heterosexuality rather than a lack of sexuality. Then I moved to the middle—a three or a four—imagining the line like a survey, its center a shrug. Neutral. No opinion. Do not care either way.

44

AT THE BEGINNING OF ELEVENTH GRADE, MY PARENTS moved an hour and a half away. I moved into the high school dorm and stopped eating. I flipped through magazines and studied the gaunt girls who stared and scowled, bored in parking lots and alleyways, bodies arranged into angles. Haunted and hunted. Unsmiling. Every image implied that there was no future other than the weight of the past. I could almost see the girls sighing. I could almost see them rolling their eyes and saying, *Whatever. Nobody cares.* Every lunch, I bought a diet lemonade and ate the ice cubes as a meal. The more weight I lost, the more my friends told me I looked great. The more the adults in my life told me I looked great. No one worried. I looked in the mirror and started to see it: Hollowed cheeks. Dead stare. Sometimes, I rolled my eyes at my reflection. *Whatever,* I mouthed. *Nobody cares.* There was so much pressure: take the hardest classes, make the highest grades. It was as if I was choreographing my own disappearing act.

The dancers said cigarettes suppressed the appetite, helped them keep pirouetting after they hadn't eaten for days. We snuck off to parking decks to smoke together, listening to Hole on the car stereo and screaming along. I wanted someone to hear and get angry. I wanted a reason and a name for the anger I felt. I didn't know how I'd ended up here. I was the girl I was, then I wasn't. Every photograph, every image I saw in a magazine seemed like a primer, a to-do list of the ways I could undo myself.

45

WHEN THE GYNECOLOGIST TOLD ME HE'D BROKEN MY hymen, I was focused very intently on ice. This was because I was chewing ice. I was in the recovery room of Women's Medical Center after my first surgery and trying not to think about my body, which would mean thinking about the pain inside of my body. So I kept chewing and thinking about ice. It was the perfect kind of ice, frozen not into cubes but into ovals the size and shape of pinkie fingernails. When I bit down, I felt a strangely electric but nonetheless perfect jolt. The ice was packed densely into a paper cup and covered with Diet Coke. The nurses said it'd help my nausea. It did not help my nausea. I held the cup with its Diet Coke and perfect pinkie-nail ice up at the level of my chin and I kept falling asleep. Just like that. With the cup raised up and an ice cube between my teeth. And because I had all that ice to think about, it was difficult to understand what the gynecologist was saying about what he'd just done inside of my body.

I did understand the general idea of what he'd done. He used several sharp instruments, guided by a camera, to cut into, inflate, and explore my lower abdomen. He'd explained the process after a full pelvic examination and Pap smear, during which he wore latex gloves and told me that I would feel a little pressure. I felt a lot of pressure. He looked up at the ceiling and the fluorescent lights that decorated it. His eyebrows pushed against each other. I felt very cold and afraid and so I looked up at the ceiling and its lights, too.

After the exam was over, he told me in his whisper-voice to get dressed and meet him in his formal office along with my mother. She had to be present during my consultations because I was a minor. His nurse smiled and blinked a few times. She rubbed my back then told me in her own whisper-voice that his office was the first room on the left. And then I was standing in the middle of the exam room. Alone, in a paper gown and with no panties on. I was just standing, in a moment of impossible quiet, until panic keened in my ears.

The Mayo Clinic recommends that women receive a full pelvic examination and Pap smear when they meet one or both of the following criteria: (1) they are twenty-one years old, and/or (2) they have been sexually active for three years. At the time of the pelvic examination and Pap smear that left me just standing, in a moment of impossible quiet, I was seventeen years old. I had not been sexually active, though I had already experienced several prior pelvic examinations, which, the Mayo Clinic's experts stressed, did not make me any less of a virgin.

In the center of the gynecologist's office sat a huge oak desk, like a giant freighter anchored on the navy blue carpet. Both the gynecologist and my mother looked at me with expectant and worried faces. On his desk stood drawings of women who stood to the front and then to the side, their skin peeled off to show the amorphous pink shapes inside. I was grateful for my clothes.

"Well," the gynecologist said, "there's an area behind your uterus called the cul-de-sac."

"Like the circle down the street that people turn their cars around in," I said.

My mother dipped her head to the side a little and said, "*Emily*," in her own whisper-voice, the one with the italics, which meant that this was not a time for joking. I stopped joking. The gynecologist pointed his pen toward one of the side-facing women. Inside of her body were three elongated pink ovals stacked on top of one another, like sunken balloons who felt sad that the party was gone.

"This is the uterus." He pointed to one of the ovals, "and this is the rectum. And here"—he moved his pen back and forth—"is the cul-de-sac, right in between them. See?" I leaned forward and nodded to indicate that I had seen. I was afraid to say it out loud. I was afraid to say yes. "I felt several spots of endometriosis there," he said, "which explains a lot of the problems you are having."

My foot tapped itself against the floor, so my mother put her hand on my knee. Her palm felt warm. I realized that I still felt very cold. I was old enough to have an open and serious conversation about the most private parts of my body, apparently, and even though I didn't actually want to participate in the conversation, I didn't want to stop it.

Endometriosis, the gynecologist explained, is a condition in which uterine tissue grows outside of the uterus, like very aggressive and insistent weeds. He couldn't explain why this happened, or what caused it to happen, or what would make it stop happening. No one could. No one knew. He couldn't explain why no one knew. He could explain that this could possibly explain why my last period had lasted almost an entire year, and the pass-out pain, and the blood and the blood and the blood. It meant I would probably have a difficult time getting pregnant. It meant that sex would probably be extremely painful.

"Do you understand what I mean?" he asked. I nodded. I was afraid to say yes. I was afraid to say that I didn't understand, that he hadn't answered any of the questions I was too afraid to ask in the first place. In that room, my body existed without me.

46

BEFORE I HAD MY FIRST LAPAROSCOPIC SURGERY, I DIDN'T know what term to use when I talked to my friends. *Laparoscopic surgery* sounded too vague and too technical. It also required follow-up details, a description of how the doctor planned to place a camera and surgical instruments inside of my body in order to figure out what had gone wrong there. *Exploratory surgery* seemed too alarming, though it was accurate and also implied a sense of adventure. I settled on *female surgery*, which was accurate and had the added bonus of stopping all follow-up questions. The surgery was the day before my senior prom. The theme was For One Night Only. I'd bought a navy blue dress with silver sparkles and strappy silver sandals, both of which stayed in my closet, unworn but still hopeful with their clearance price tags, for four years before I gave them to the Goodwill.

At the time of my first surgery, I was nowhere near sexually active. The closest I had ever come to being anywhere near sexually active happened when I walked the track circling Joe Tucker Park with my kind-of-boyfriend, a visual arts major at my high school. I attempted to hold my kind-of-boyfriend's hand, but his hands were too sweaty and my hands were too cold. Kind-of-boyfriend and I stopped walking and started standing on a small spot of green past the swing sets and slides, beneath an ancient, stubborn pine tree that no one dared to cut down. I attempted to move my lips the way women in the movies move their lips when they want to be kissed.

"Are you okay?" kind-of-boyfriend asked me, so I swanned out my neck so my lips almost met his. He did not respond in kind. He said, "People might see us," and I said "So?" I closed my eyes and waited. Nothing happened. I opened my eyes to see kind-of-boyfriend shake his head as a gray-haired woman with an actual Walkman walked past, without even once looking at us.

In the recovery room, I kept chewing ice as the gynecologist listed all the places he'd found endometriosis—in the cul-de-sac, as he'd predicted, and under my right ovary, and on my right ovary, and inside my right ovary—during which I heard mostly *crunch crunch crunch.* I was getting into a rhythm with it, a strange little song of sorts. Then he told me that he'd broken my hymen. I kept chewing. He told me not to worry, that he had sewn my hymen up again. Good as new. I stopped chewing. The hand holding the cup of ice fell. My mother grabbed the cup before it fell, too.

"Whoopsie," she said.

"What?" I said, my voice thick with drugs and cold.

"I repaired it," the gynecologist said. He smiled broadly. "I sewed it up, so don't worry."

"*Why?*" my mother asked.

"What do you mean, you sewed it up?"

"Just that," he said. "I repaired it."

"*Why?*" my mother repeated. "If you'd left it broken, you'd just be doing her a favor."

"I didn't even think that was possible?" My voice made an upturn at the end, turning it into a question. The gynecologist nodded in assent. He smiled even more broadly. He looked so proud of himself. I didn't want to disappoint him. He moved on to talk about how and when and where I could shower. I was still holding my hand in a *C* shape right below my chin, so my mother put the cup of ice back in my hand. I looked at her face as a way to gauge how I should respond, but her face wasn't giving any hints. I wanted to ask him why he'd sewn up my hymen, but I also wanted to be a good patient. I nodded my thanks and started chewing ice again, focusing on the noise instead of what had happened to my hymen while I was on the surgical table, asleep.

In ancient Greece, Hymen was a male, though he was not a male human being. He was a male god and his duties required him to attend every wedding ceremony. He was tremendously busy. In sculptures and paintings and other artistic representations, he's shown wearing a garland of flowers and carrying a torch.

The Wikipedia page for Hymen (god) offers a link to Hymen (disambiguation) and a photograph of George Rennie's sculpture titled *Cupid Rekindling the Torch of Hymen*. In Rennie's sculpture, Hymen indeed sports a garland of flowers, along with a penis, which indicates that he is (1) a male and (2) a male who is confident about his sexuality. He also indeed carries a torch, though it doesn't look like a torch. It looks like a vibrator. It looks so much like a vibrator that upon seeing the photograph of the sculpture, I said to myself and my cats and out loud, "Is that a *vibrator*?"

Neither myself nor my cats answered.

47

I CELEBRATED MY EIGHTEENTH BIRTHDAY BY TAKING AN AP Calculus exam. It was not a test that I wanted to take. I could opt out of only one AP exam and I'd chosen to skip the AP Economics test, much to my econ-major father's disappointment. He'd tried to help me as I muddled through Adam Smith and John Maynard Keynes, as I tried to understand the metaphors our teacher gave us.

"But if the government is in debt," I said, "why not just make more money?"

"Because then the money would be worthless," my father said, patiently.

"Just split the money evenly among everyone, then."

My father shook his head. "That's called communism, and it's not a bad idea. It's just not going to help you on this test."

My "female problems" had already returned. I was so worried I wouldn't be able to function in the physical sense that I didn't worry about the fact that I still wasn't entirely sure what the word *function* meant in the mathematical sense. On the morning of the exam, I started my period. I took two Wygesic and a Phenergan. It was the only way I could sit upright without vomiting for three hours and fifteen minutes.

I scored a one out of five on my practice exam. I scored a three out of five on my official exam.

•

Approximately four months after my first operation, I sat in the gynecologist's office, again, looking at his giant freighter of an oak desk while my foot tapped itself against the carpet. My mother sat beside me. She did not put her hand on my knee to make my foot stop tapping itself. Instead, she asked the gynecologist why all my pain never seemed to stop. She was no longer using her whisper-voice. The gynecologist explained that my endometriosis had grown back. He used the word *aggressive*. Neither he nor any other doctor could explain exactly why my endometriosis had grown back, and aggressively, because neither he nor any other doctor knew why anyone's endometriosis grew, whether aggressively or gently, in the first place.

The gynecologist said it was time for more aggressive measures. It was time for more aggressive surgery. It was time for more aggressive hormones. After my next operation, I was to start receiving Lupron Depot injections, which would prevent my body from producing estrogen. I would at that point enter a medically induced menopausal state.

"That stuff you wanted me to take?" My mother shook her head. "No way."

When she tells the story, my mother adds this: at this point, I was no longer a minor, which meant that she had no authority when it came to my medical care.

My mother stresses this point: It was my decision to begin treatment with Lupron. It was my choice.

My mother is correct, of course, but I also stress this point: I had no choice.

Had I refused to take Lupron, my insurance company would've refused to pay for any future surgeries, as I would've refused to try nonsurgical options first.

"Do you understand?" The gynecologist asked. I nodded. I did not understand. He handed me a pamphlet about the drug's side effects. He handed me another pamphlet about menopausal symptoms.

The women on the cover differed from the usual drawings on his pamphlets. They got to keep their skin, over which they wore cardigan twinsets and gray grandmother hair and prune-mouthed expressions of concern. In a few weeks, I would move to New York to become a first-year student at Sarah Lawrence. I would say *first-year* and not *freshman*, emphatically. I would pack my Birkenstocks, my love bead necklaces, my cat's-eye ring, my favorite sweaters, my Tori Amos poster, my Lupron injections, my pain pills, my anti-nausea pills, my antidepressants, and an ice pack for when the hot flashes got too bad.

48

My mother does not like it when I talk and/or write about Lupron. Or rather, my mother does not like the way that I talk and/or write about Lupron.

"What you need to do," my mother says, "is just tell your *personal* story of your *personal* experience with Lupron. Then, no one can come back on you." She doesn't want me to use the names of hospitals. She doesn't want me to use the names of doctors. There will be consequences, she says—not for the hospitals and/or doctors, but for me.

"That's fine," I say, "because I can't imagine anything much worse than the consequences I've already faced. Can you?"

I don't wait for an answer. I already know.

On April 9, 1985, the FDA approved a drug for the treatment of prostate cancer—which means, of course, that it was approved as a drug intended for male bodies. In its various forms, this drug would come to be known as: leuprolide acetate, leuprolide acetate for depot suspension, Lupron, Lupron Depot, leuprolide, Lupron Depot-Ped, Eligard, Viadur, Leuprolide (intradermal route, intramuscular route, subcutaneous route), and Lupron injection (for daily subcutaneous injection).

The drug treats prostate cancer like this: After the medicine has been injected, it moves to the pituitary gland, where it finds the gonadotropin-releasing hormone receptor, or the GnRHR. The GnRHR's job is to catch the gonadotropin-releasing hormone, or GnRH, after it's released from the hypothalamus. GnRH tells other cells in the pituitary gland to release the luteinizing hormone, also known as lutropin, which tells the testicles to produce testosterone. Lupron and other GnRH antagonists interrupt this process by, in a manner of speaking, antagonizing the GnRHRs. The drug creates a chain of nonreactions: If the GnRH receptor doesn't catch GnRH, it can't release lutropin, which means the testicles can't produce testosterone. When the testicles stop producing testosterone, the owner of said testicles is chemically castrated. The growth of tumors in his prostate slows.

But male bodies aren't the only bodies that produce lutropin. In female bodies, lutropin encourages the ovaries to produce estrogen. If a female receives a Lupron injection, she enters chemically induced menopause. This could, metaphorically, be called female castration.

Doctors had a theory: If estrogen feeds the growth of endometrial tissue inside of the uterus, wouldn't it also feed the growth of endometrial tissue outside of the uterus? And if a woman's estrogen levels were reduced to an extreme degree, wouldn't that also reduce the growth of endometriosis?

On January 26, 1989, the FDA approved a new form of Lupron—Lupron Depot (leuprolide acetate for depot suspension)—as a treatment for advanced prostate cancer. It was also approved as a treatment for endometriosis.

According to the American Cancer Society, 2.9 million American men live with prostate cancer diagnoses. More than 7 million American women have been diagnosed with endometriosis.

The FDA's approval of Lupron gave countless women, many of whom had been raised not to talk openly about endometriosis and other aspects of their reproductive health, hope.

It also gave the pharmaceutical company millions of potential patients afraid and ashamed to openly talk about the disease their medication treated, much less the treatment itself.

A few days into my recovery from my second surgery, my mother's best friend, a nurse, came to our house with a Lupron injection and some heavy-duty gloves. She took the injection out of its packaging. She flicked the side of the syringe until the particulates had dispersed. I saw my mother wince. She still stayed in the room, holding my hand.

"I'm sorry," my mother's best friend said as the needle went in, as she pushed in the plunger, as the liquid and the particulates made their way into my body. "I'm sorry, Emily. I'm so sorry."

For three days, it was impossible to sit or to lie on the side of the injection site.

This was the least painful of my Lupron injections.

49

In late August 1998, I began my freshman year of college. I was still recovering from surgery, which meant I wasn't supposed to exert myself. I sat on my twin bed while my father unpacked the Moody Blues CDs I'd borrowed/stolen from him, my mandala-in-the-sky poster, my three-month supply of Prozac. I watched my roommate unpack her Serge Gainsbourg CDs, her Truffaut poster, her French cigarettes. I mouthed to my father, *Help*.

My mother walked around campus with a Lupron injection in her purse. She needed to find the health services building so that she could hand over the injection—along with its lengthy packet of precautions and cautions for the safety of the injector and the injectee. The nurses pursed their lips, scratched the scalps beneath their bangs. They seemed to dread giving the injection every bit as much as I dreaded getting it.

In November of my freshman year, I came home early for Thanksgiving break so that I could see the gynecologist, and as soon as possible.

Here is what happened: I woke one morning to see that my lower abdomen was purple. Violet. Darkly, unmistakably so. And I hadn't fallen or stumbled or walked drunk-blind into anything, so I headed to health services. The nurses were deeply concerned. They were also deeply confused. They pursed their lips, scratched their scalps. They knew that blood had pooled under my skin and become a hematoma, but they didn't know how. Neither did the physician at the near-est emergency room. No one would know, they said, until someone looked inside of my body.

At the airport, my mother pulled me into the first bathroom we passed.

"Show me what you're talking about," she said. I bent down and looked under the row of stalls and saw they were all empty.

"All clear," I said, so we walked into the same stall. I unbuttoned and pulled down the right side of my jeans.

My mother took in a long, hissing breath. "Je-s-us," she said. She made the word three syllables with another hiss of breath at the end.

"It's better than it was," I said.

"I wouldn't call that better," she said.

I shrugged and buttoned my jeans. "You get used to things, I guess."

50

A FEW DAYS BEFORE THANKSGIVING OF MY FRESHMAN YEAR, the gynecologist told me that my endometriosis had grown back. Again. Aggressively. I was no longer a minor and because we already knew what everyone would say, my mother stayed in the waiting room while I sat in the gynecologist's office, head bobbing on the waves of the pain medication I had to take in order to walk.

When the gynecologist looked inside of my body for the third time, he found a large endometrioma—a cyst comprised of endometrial tissue filled with blood—on my appendix. He also found evidence that other endometriomas had recently burst on and around the area. Since the blood in endometriomas is typically brown, the gynecologist referred to them as chocolate milk cysts.

My college friends all seemed to spend a great deal of their time doing three things: (1) talking about how badly they needed to get laid, (2) getting laid, and (3) talking about how badly they needed to get laid again. I didn't spend any of my time doing any of those three things. All the pamphlets about menopause said I should discuss a decreased sex drive with a doctor. So I decided to discuss my absent sex drive with this doctor at one of my postsurgical appointments.

"I'm just a little worried because I don't want to have sex," I said.

"Do you mean that you're not sexually attracted to *men*?"

"No," I said, "I mean that I'm not sexually attracted to *anyone*."

The gynecologist said, "Hm." It was the kind of *hm* that indicated he didn't believe my italics. That he instead believed I wasn't sexually attracted to *men*, which indicated that I was sexually attracted to *women* and was ashamed of it.

By the time I had started my period, most of my classmates began to experience sexual feelings. By the year after that, I realized that I was not.

All of this was awkward.

All of this was especially awkward because I didn't have the language for it, didn't have the right words to explain.

I looked at the boys. I looked at the girls. And I felt nothing.

A 2015 study found that 74 percent of women who say they are not interested in engaging in sexual contact with other women were nonetheless aroused by images of naked women. By the time of my third surgery, I had engaged in sexual contact with another female zero times, unless you count awkward kissing during very awkward games of spin the bottle on the floor of my resident adviser's dorm room.

The study makes no mention of games of spin the bottle, awkward or otherwise.

51

"So," Leia asked, "you've really, like, never done it? Like, *ever?*"

It was a Saturday, just around noon. By some miracle, my best friend and I had managed to make it down the hill to the campus dining hall in time to indulge in our deepest obsession: the weekend waffle bar. And perhaps because I was granted this great fortune, I was not granted the great fortune of avoiding yet another conversation about the fact that I was not, had never been, and honestly really did not plan to be sexually active. I'd tried to not tell her, but she guessed anyway.

That wasn't difficult.

While my classmates were engaging in sexual activities in one another's dorm rooms, I sat in my room alone, eating dry Lucky Charms straight from the box while listening to Tori Amos. Even though I called Leia my best friend, it was difficult to talk to her about my sexual activities or the lack thereof. It was difficult to talk to her about anything that had to do with the body, my body especially, since her body was beautiful. In her tweens and early teens, she'd worked as a model, shuffling her way through the shoving subway crowds after school, finding the right light in photo shoot after photo shoot. I always knew, somehow, that our friendship was temporary: after graduation, I'd fly back south to live in some sweaty nowhere, and she'd stay in New York, making her beautiful way through the subways. The fact that I knew that soon I wouldn't see her face-to-face again made it somewhat easier to talk to her about the body, my body, and its lack of sexual activities.

I shook my head. "Never," I said. "Like, never ever. Like, never ever even close, actually." Her mouth was too full of waffles for her to make words, so she moved her head very slowly to one side and another, as if she were saying *no, no*, as if she were saying *in no way do I agree*.

"Aren't you, like, *dying?*"

I shook my head like she'd shaken hers. *No*, I wanted to say. *In no way am I, like, dying. I am, like, the absolute opposite of dying. I have never really wanted to do it, like ever, which isn't anything like dying except in that, like death, it's confusing.* I looked down at the napkin in my lap and my hands on top of the napkin. Almost all my fingernails, which I'd painted flame red, were bare. I couldn't remember how that had happened.

52

AFTER A WHILE THE GYNECOLOGIST WAS EITHER CONVINCED that (1) I did not, in fact, mean that I was attracted to *women* instead of *men* or that (2) if I *was* attracted to *women* instead of *men*, I wasn't going to tell him about it, even if my mother wasn't in the room. And so he said, "Think about it this way," and I said, "Okay." I prepared to think about it this way. I wanted to be a good patient.

"Imagine you are drowning," the gynecologist said, and so I began to imagine that I was drowning. This wasn't very difficult because I actually had, at age four, almost drowned, so I was actually remembering drowning instead of imagining drowning. I thought of all the water in all the forms I'd seen: the bright white-blue of my aunt's overchlorinated aboveground pool. The Hudson River, a muddy stripe on the ground that turned blue as my airplane began its final descent into New York. The snow that gathered itself in thick piles, hiding my college campus's thin, leafless bushes. I imagined the snow melting, the sides of my aunt's pool collapsing, the Hudson River overflowing its banks. I imagined all that water flowing together while I floated just below its surface. I imagined myself looking up at the waves from the other side, watching them gather and fade away, a pattern that repeated endlessly.

The gynecologist kept talking: "As you drown, your systems go, one by one, according to what the body needs most. Your digestion stops, your breathing stops, and then your heart stops, and your brain stops last, because that's what your body needs most." I imagined my digestion and my breathing stopping, one by one, until I was just a heart and a brain, and then just a brain.

"Right now," the gynecologist said, "you are drowning." I didn't argue. "What does your body need least? Sex. So your sex drive has shut down."

So I had never actually stopped drowning. I'd been walking around all this time, drowning. And no one who is drowning is also thinking, *Perhaps this is the right time for me to engage in sexual intercourse.* It made a lot of sense, so I said, "That makes a lot of sense."

What I didn't say: Actual drowning was a lot better than the metaphorical drowning I had experienced, all this time, walking around. Actual drowning was kind of pleasant. Everything was soft and blue, even the light. I felt very peaceful.

Wikipedia notes that even if a drowning person tries to hold her breath, her body will try to breathe, despite herself, as a reflex.

When I was an actually-really-drowning person, I did not hold my breath. I don't think my body tried to breathe, either. I didn't feel like I needed to breathe at all, which was a relief. While I was metaphorically drowning—which is what I had been doing, apparently, all this time—I always needed to breathe, which was unpleasant. Even breathing hurt. So I walked around in my Birkenstocks and ordered egg sandwiches and talked about *The History of the Peloponnesian War* and drowned metaphorically.

Sometimes I stopped and reminded myself to breathe. Then I would breathe in shallow, rhythmic melodies. Sometimes I remembered how my fifth-grade teacher had told us to count our breaths, and then I'd feel myself stop breathing. I tried to forget. Sometimes I wished that my breathing would do its own thing and just stop, by its own volition. Sometimes I wanted nothing more than to have my own breathing just stop.

When I was actually-really-drowning, things were much nicer. I just hung there, in the water, which was very warm, feeling relaxed. I didn't even have to breathe. It was that easy, drowning. It was that easy.

53

IN MAY OF MY FRESHMAN YEAR, I ATTENDED A BELTANE ceremony to celebrate summer and sun and returning warmth, growth and abundance and protection, and those three things which, for me, felt most mysterious: desire, pleasure, and well-functioning fertility. Instead of a dress, I wore a pink-and-white slip I found at the thrift store in the hospital's basement. Instead of focusing on intentions or the elements or the moon, I worried about the bonfire building itself in the center of our circle. I worried that a flame would escape and ignite my slip. It was probably 97 percent rayon, and therefore probably 97 percent flammable.

When it was my turn to jump over the fire, I held my skirt up and close to my legs. I closed my eyes. I expected to burn. When I opened my eyes, I stood safely on the other side, consumed by nothing more dangerous than relief. In the moment, it felt enough like what people call pleasure.

Flushed and flaming with a courage stoked from standing outside in the still-cold May night, the circle dissolved and recircled in an on-campus apartment. We passed a bottle of vodka until it emptied, then refilled it with the damiana liqueur we'd made with another bottle of vodka. It tasted like sweet tea and rubbing alcohol and the dandelion fluff that blows back into your mouth when you blow it away with your wish. Sarah said it was a love potion, that it would make anyone feel sexy. Horny. Full of desire. She said all three things, just like that, as if to differentiate between and order them. I took the bottle and leaned my head back. I gulped. I wanted to feel sexy. I wanted to feel horny. I wanted to understand what it meant, to be full of desire.

54

THERE WAS A BOY IN THE BELTANE CIRCLE WHO WASN'T actually a boy. He was a man who said he'd spent his early twenties jumping out of helicopters on military missions. He looked like Marlon Brando and had visions of the Green Man after parachuting into forests. "Except they weren't actually visions," he said. "One minute I was looking at a circle of leaves, and then he was there. He was actually *there.*" He smelled like Old Spice and nag champa. I decided to try to be in love with him.

That Beltane, after we'd sent the spirits and the fire we built for them on their ways, after we had eaten spaghetti out of the giant silver pot because there were no bowls, after we'd drunk all the vodka and damiana liqueur and red wine, after Bella threw up so hard that a spaghetti noodle came out of her nose, I stumbled back to the Military Man's dorm room. He pushed Play on the CD player then sashayed into the bathroom.

I sat on his navy duvet cover and listened to the organ music, funereal and ghostly, at the beginning of "A Whiter Shade of Pale." I realized I was very drunk. I wasn't sitting still. I was *attempting* to sit still, an act that required an enormous amount of concentration. Still, I recognized that something major was about to happen. "It was *so* major," I imagined myself saying to Leia later. I practiced saying it, silently. I held the *so* like a very long note.

When the Military Man came out of the bathroom, he wasn't wearing the jeans and the white T-shirt he'd worn to jump over the fire. Instead, he wore a terry cloth bathrobe, so old that the belt frayed unrecognizably at the ends. Then he wasn't wearing the bathrobe. I looked at the broad, smooth expanse of his shaved chest. I looked down. He was wearing a pair of blue boxer shorts with a cartoon Tigger on them, paws splayed into jazz hands, mouth split into a grin as if to say, *Surprise.* When the Military Man turned around, Tigger turned around with him. I saw Tigger's tail on his rear end. The Military Man turned back to me and splayed his fingers like Tigger's. *Surprise.* I imagined myself as the self who existed after this moment had ended, as the self telling Leia what had happened in the moment I thought was going to be so major. I replaced the *so* with *not.*

"*Prrrrrrrrrr,*" he said, rolling his tongue like my grammar school Spanish teacher did. I waited for the rest of the word—*Pirata? Presente? Privado? Prisa?* But there wasn't a rest of the word, just a *prrrrrrrrrr.*

I put my hand on my purse. "It's getting late."

He shook his head and wiggled his finger, left to right. And then he was kissing me. I might have been kissing him. I thought about the fire. How it made everyone look beautiful. How looking at everyone's beauty was a pleasure I could understand.

I also thought about Tigger.

"Okay," I said, pushing him backward, gently, with one hand against his hairless chest. "But nothing but kissing."

He nodded and wiggled his finger again, back and forth, at the same rate.

Perhaps because of that night and its ceremony and beauty, perhaps because he had gulped down even more vodka than me, we both kept the agreement. Nothing but kissing. I stayed in his room, falling in and out of sleep, of a dream about a building full of stairs that never ended or reached anything.

When I walked from his dorm in the morning, I kept my head high. I wanted to give the impression of triumph, of someone who'd awakened in a bed of her own wrinkled dress and walked away, leaving her cherry behind.

55

MANY OF MY COLLEGE FRIENDS REMAINED CONCERNED about my lack of sexual activities. It was, like, so 1950s. It was, like, so repressive, so dire. It was one of those things you just had to *get over with*. One night, Leia decided to start at the beginning.

"I am going to teach you how to flirt." She sipped out of a red Solo cup sloshing with red wine. She swayed and ashed a cigarette out of my open dorm room window. "We'll do it like a class. You fucking love class."

I nodded, emphatically, keeping my lips just above the lip of my own sloshing red Solo cup. "Yes. I fucking love that. I fucking love class." In other words: I remembered that learning from experience is just one way of learning. In other words: I remembered that the reason I fucking loved class was that, in class, I was in control. I fucking loved class because it gave me a vocabulary that allowed me to at least fake understanding, even if I didn't understand the subject completely.

And so Leia set up a double date involving herself, a friend she was thinking about dating, myself, and her friend's older brother. We ate dinner in a Japanese restaurant where everything looked shockingly white-white. We drank warm sake out of small wooden boxes. They ate pink slivers of fish, layered like scales over rice. I ate the rice. I was nervous, and though the sake tasted a little like peroxide, I knew that if I drank enough I'd forget the taste, and then I'd forget to be nervous. It was the way I'd learned to fake it, to pretend I was a person who knew any part of what she should do.

By the time Leia and our dates walked out of the restaurant and into the steam heat of the city, everything—the street signs and strangers and cabbies clicking off their OCCUPIED signs in perfect coordination—looked at us in kindness. All the lights were hazy-perfect. I smiled without worrying that I had anything in my teeth. My friend moved closer to her friend, and both of them loud-laughed in a way that implied that they may soon have successful sex. Her friend's older brother was an actor, which he thought would make me sexually attracted to him. He was not correct. But he did mention my favorite play—Anton Chekhov's *The Cherry Orchard*—which made me feel an interest that seemed significant enough for me to call it attraction. It also made me want to talk.

I was telling him how much I loved the part in act 4 where Lyubov tells the trees and the house and her youth goodbye, when Leia took my hand. I thought she meant the gesture in a happy-fun way, in a *we are both very drunk so let's hold hands and laugh and maybe, if we are drunk enough but not too drunk, we could skip for a few steps* kind of way. Then she pulled my hand and me sharply to the left.

She was not feeling happy-fun-skipping-drunk. "What are you *doing*," Leia said, and I said, "What," and she said, "Why are you *talking* about *The* Cherry *Orchard*," just like that, with all those italics and no question mark at the end.

I said, with a careful question mark, "Because I like *The Cherry Orchard*?" I meant to indicate both that I did not understand why she was asking me this question and that I was no longer sure if liking *The Cherry Orchard* was an appropriate thing to do.

"You are supposed to be *flirting*," she said, with the italics and no contraction, and I said, "I am?" I meant to indicate that I assumed I was already flirting, not that I didn't know I was supposed to be flirting. It occurred to me that perhaps the boys could be listening, perhaps they could hear it, this conversation about how I was not doing what one should be doing when *flirting*. I looked over at them and saw them lost in their private laughter, in their nods and back thumps and gestures.

"Flirting does not involve talking about *The* Cherry *Orchard*," she said, letting my hand go and sending me stumbling toward her friend's brother with an aggravated finality. And suddenly the streets and their lights and their sounds seemed strange and threatening, like the city and all its cars and lights and weather had descended into a slow but emphatic hiss.

56

I FIRST READ DAVID MAMET'S ADAPTATION OF *THE CHERRY Orchard* when I was in seventh grade. I liked the play a great deal because everyone had complicated names and no one ever knew what to do about their trees or their land or their fur hats or anything. Mamet also wrote an introduction to the play, and in it he explained what he thought Chekhov meant: that this wasn't really a play about forestry or real estate or the collapse of the Russian aristocracy. This was a play about sexual frustration, and honestly about little else.

I had little idea what sexual frustration was, actually or approximately. Still, the term was thrilling. I spent three weeks practicing different ways to say it in my oral book report. I prayed that I wouldn't freak out and miss my chance to say *sex* for a totally legitimate reason in front of the coolest kids in my class. Then I prayed that God would forgive me for praying about something like that. I told myself to imagine I was back at the beach with Mary while her mother was at the pool, which meant we could say words like *sex* and *orgasm* and laugh as much as we wanted, or even play the game that consisted entirely of saying the word *penis*, first in a whisper, then moving slowly up in volume until you had to scream penis or forfeit the game. I told myself to be brave. I told myself I'd never forfeit the game.

57

I DID NOT END UP LOSING MY VIRGINITY TO MY FRIEND'S
friend's brother. I saw him one more time for one single official date, in
someone else's Brooklyn brownstone, while the cat he was cat-sitting
stared angrily from the corner. It didn't take me long to discover that,
Chekhov aside, I had far more in common with the cat. We drank
red wine out of old jelly jars and made out perfunctorily. Neither
the actor nor the cat seemed impressed. When his hand slipped into
the waistband of my jeans, I stopped kissing him. At first, he didn't
notice, so I made an *um* noise and pulled my lips away.

"What's the problem?" He sent an exasperated puff of air through
his lips, which were rimmed red with wine like lipstick, which, The
Learning Channel had told me, symbolized sexual maturity. There,
on that couch, I didn't feel as though I had reached sexual maturity.
I felt definitively not sexually mature enough to have the actor's hand
in my pants.

"Can we slow down? I think I need to slow down." The actor
pushed out another little puff of air before he took his hand and his
lips away.

We sat on the couch for a few minutes, pretending we had anything to talk about, before I said it was getting late. He agreed. He
walked me to the train station. We smoked cigarettes so we wouldn't
have to talk. Before I walked into the station and toward the train
that would take me away, he said that he'd forgotten something. He'd
bought me a Christmas present: a copy of Rilke's *Letters to a Young*

Poet, which he'd wrapped in baby blue paper. It was the third time I'd received the book as a gift. I pretended that I was excited to read it, that it was the absolute most perfect thing. I hugged him and held my face in such a way as to indicate, I hoped, that I would be amenable to one last kiss.

He would not kiss me.

I took the train back to campus, reading through Rilke's answers and trying to imagine the questions he was asked.

I did not reapply my lipstick.

58

In a letter written not long after he was married, Rilke describes love between two people in terms of a limitation that hinders one's freedom. For Rilke, love in its purest form has nothing to do with the body, or with the people who live inside of those bodies. Instead, love is something we find only when we find solitude, when we learn not just to love the other but to love the distance between us. Then, we recognize the wonder of the vast space in which we live. We recognize that vast, empty space itself as love, and from this distance only, we can best know and love one another.

I never heard from the actor again. I rewrapped *Letters to a Young Poet* in that same blue paper and slipped it onto a high shelf in my closet, like a time capsule of a version of myself I'd already learned to forget. A few months after our only date, I realized I'd left it behind as I sat in an airport, listening for the gate announcement. It was time to fly away from New York. I felt peace. I felt ready to let the plane take me up and away and into that vast blue, the everything that is empty space.

59

BY THE END OF MY SOPHOMORE YEAR IN COLLEGE, I'D HAD A total of four laparoscopic surgeries for the express purpose of seeking out and removing growths of endometrial tissue in my abdomen. Prior to the first and second laparoscopic surgeries, I had not yet had my first kiss. Prior to the first, second, third, and fourth laparoscopic surgeries, I had not engaged in sexual intercourse of any kind. Even though I had had many Pap smears and pelvic exams, I was, according to the Mayo Clinic, still a virgin. During the first and second laparoscopic surgeries, the surgeon tore my hymen membrane, which he repaired with small sutures in a procedure known as a hymenorrhaphy.

Prior to none of these procedures did I express a wish that, should my hymen be torn, it should be sewn back up.

After both of these procedures, I told my mother that I wished he would've left my hymen broken, that I could've just gotten it over with in that way. She emphatically agreed.

Many assume that if a female person's hymen is not intact, that female person is no longer a virgin. According to Wikipedia, many heterosexuals consider themselves virgins until they engage in sexual intercourse involving penile-vaginal penetration. In other words, many heterosexuals consider themselves virgins until they have made it through all the bases and achieved a home run. The act of sliding into home presumably pierces the hymen, which, in most cases, causes only minimal pain and bleeding.

However, only 43 percent of women bleed the first time they engage in sexual intercourse. This indicates that when 57 percent of women first engage in sexual intercourse, their hymens are not intact. The hymen may not have been present in the body from birth; alternately, it may have been broken during physical exercise, such as a softball game or cheerleading.

I'm not sure if I was saving my cherry for marriage or not. I am sure that I didn't think about my cherry the way that my friends did. They described it as something uncomfortable, poisonous, like a boil that needs to be lanced. They talked about virginity in the past tense, but sex was always in the present. They talked about being so turned on and so horny and so hard up and every time, I could only think of other nouns that could be described by those adjectives: Light switch. Armadillo. Eggs.

"I know," I would say, "I just need to, like, *do It*."

I did not know.

My mother sometimes spoke and with a kind of pre–Vatican II intensity about how *It* should not happen until you have been lawfully married in the eyes of God in an actual church, or at least when you are engaged. I listened and nodded and promised, just like I listened and nodded and promised when she spoke with a pre–Vatican II intensity about how I shouldn't drink to excess, smoke marijuana or tobacco cigarettes, or wear so damn much black eyeliner. The promise I made her about *It*, however, was the promise I came closest to meaning.

And it did seem like an easy excuse, an easy reason, an easy way to talk about the way I didn't feel about sexual intercourse. The more time passed, the more it seemed feasible, the more I started telling my friends, *I've held on to it this long, so why not? It's accreted a different kind of meaning.* My friends made confused but solemn nods. Only rarely did someone say *cock tease.* A little less rarely did someone say *frigid.* Most of the time, I got away with *freak,* which felt enough like being spared.

60

HERE IS WHERE I WOULD LIKE TO END THE STORY, LEAVING it neatly packaged, tied and bowed and wrapped in pale blue paper. Or else, here is where I would like to insert the kind of twist around which stories are built: that I, perhaps, wasn't attracted to the actor because I was attracted instead to his brother, or to Leia. But this story isn't built around a resolution so much as the strange insistence that something was missing in me, in my body.

I didn't understand why one person's body would thrum with passion in the presence of another person's body because I had never experienced it, any of it: passion, attraction, lust, desire. I could only imagine what that would feel like. The way feet feel an organ's low notes through the floor of a cathedral. The way glass cracks in pleasure when struck with high-pitched notes. I was pretty sure that whatever had passed between the actor and me and the wine on the couch of that Brooklyn brownstone was nothing close to attraction. But I also didn't know, exactly, that there existed a connection between attraction and love, that for most people, love could not be True Love if attraction wasn't present.

The actor's body didn't thrum in the presence of my body. I knew that. But because I didn't experience that thrum in the presence of any body, I didn't know that this meant, for him, that we couldn't be in love. I didn't know that I shouldn't take the gift or the fact that he had wrapped it, so carefully and in such beautifully blue paper, as a sign that we were meant to be together. I didn't know that parting from one single official date without a good-night kiss was a good sign that there'd be no follow-up date. How foolish I must have seemed, to leave him one and then two and then three voice mails, to send him one and then two and then three emails, to check my voice mail and inbox in the unflagging hope that I'd find a message from him. I imagined standing with him in the New York City streets, hearing the hum of idling taxicabs, watching the snow throw itself through the streetlights and shivering both with the cold and with the feeling that everything was beautiful, including us and our separate lives that could—so easily, I thought—merge into the singular.

61

WHEN MY TWICE-REPAIRED HYMEN DID BREAK, IT WAS NOT in the process of penile-vaginal penetration (a.k.a.: a home run) but instead on second base. I was twenty-four years old. The pain and bleeding was not minimal, either, but extreme and also humiliating, and therefore play stopped before any other bases were reached. In baseball terms, this experience was roughly equivalent to a force-out.

Of the hymen, Alfred Kinsey wrote: "I think any creator who claims that he had a purpose in creating the hymen certainly shows himself incapable of having done a good job." Not only did my hymen not break in the process of penile-vaginal penetration, but the associated pain and bleeding were so extreme and also humiliating that I did not get any closer to penile-vaginal penetration for quite some time. It is unclear if this proves or disproves Kinsey's remark about any creator's purpose in creating the hymen, or the doctor's purpose in twice-repairing my hymen.

62

I NEVER TOLD THE GYNECOLOGIST THAT I WAS ANGRY WITH him for performing two hymenorrhaphies without my asking him to. I never told him that I blamed the two hymenorrhaphies, and therefore him, for the extreme pain, bleeding, and humiliation I experienced when my hymen broke. I washed the blood off my legs, my arms, my hands. I pulled the bloody sheets off of my bed. I was angry as I folded them before I put them in a trash bag, as I pulled the pillow out of the bloody-handprinted pillowcase. I was angry as I saw bloody handprints on the pillow, too, and as I put both the pillow and the pillowcase into the trash bag, and as I walked to the dumpster, as I clenched my teeth and said *don't cry don't cry* to myself, as I held my nose and slid the metal door open and put the trash bag in the dumpster, as I walked back, as I clenched my teeth harder and harder. I was angry as I drove to Target and as I stood in the checkout line with a cart full of new sheets, a new pillow, Clorox bleach, overnight Kotex, and a bottle of red wine. I was angry at my silence, at my own teenage obedience, how I'd wanted to be a good patient at all times, no matter what that meant. I was at the same time angry that the gynecologist was the best doctor I'd ever had, the doctor who treated me best, who listened most and cared most and responded most, who believed me the most and tried the most to mend the goddamn mess that was my body. I was angry with the goddamn mess that was my body.

I was angry.

I was angry.

63

I FIRST EXPERIENCED PENILE-VAGINAL PENETRATION, OR made it to home base, when I was twenty-five and with a man I'd fallen in love with in an Irish bar in graduate school, where we drank straight whiskey and fed a jukebox quarters until it played nothing but Prince songs for two hours. One night while Prince rode the horn riff into the chorus of "Sexy MF," I listened as the man told me about a video he'd seen on public television as a child: a fox curled up in the grass, its body caught in time-lapsed decay. He'd never stopped thinking about it, just like I'd never stopped thinking about it, and I decided that decaying fox was as good a sign as any that this was the man I should love and date and marry.

I knew that it was supposed to hurt, that first time, so I didn't say anything about it hurting. I kept moving the way I'd seen women move in movies. I kept making the kind of noises that I'd heard women make in movies. I'd been studying for a long time, and so I tried to make my body do what my body was supposed to do. I tried to make my body say: *This is pleasurable, I am enjoying this act.* I tried to make my body into the body he and his careful kindness deserved. I wanted to be what he deserved.

I kept my eyes closed so I wouldn't have to see anything or accidentally cry, because even though he was very careful and gentle and kind, it hurt. It hurt in that white light kind of way, in that blinding and unbelievable kind of way. It hurt in that white blinding light kind of way that made everything seem unbelievable, especially that a human being could feel pain like that and still be alive, and still be a human being.

I lay there and imagined that I was somewhere else. I imagined that my body belonged to someone who definitively and absolutely was not me, and I was just kind of standing next to the bed, looking at the two of us and thinking, *That body is in so much pain. That body is in so much pain that it must not even feel like pain anymore.* And the woman who existed in my body moved the way they did in the movies. She made the right sounds and pretended to feel the right things. She had studied, and her studying paid off.

It was, I hoped, a spectacular performance.

SOME OF WHICH MAY NOT BE REVERSIBLE

64

A FEW DAYS BEFORE I STARTED EVERY PERIOD, I WANTED TO die. I wanted to die in an actual, real way, not in a metaphorical way, as in *I missed lunch, so I'm dying of hunger*; *I'm dying of boredom*; *I will die if I do not get those gorgeous shoes.* I would lie in bed and think to myself, in a nonmetaphorical way, that things would be much better for myself and, more importantly, for everyone who knew me if I just died. And then there I was again, on the balcony of my grandparents' condo at the beach, sobbing and snotting and staring down at the pier and the crabbers and their traps, tipping headfirst toward that darkness. This time, there was no hand to pull me back from it.

When I was in my midtwenties, I addressed this question with a gynecologist. Once. "I just get so depressed every time I'm about to start," I told him. I was careful not to mention the fact that I also thought about just dying so I wouldn't seem like a danger to myself or to others.

"You might have PMDD," he said. He didn't tell me what that meant or even what those letters stood for. He just hung the suggestion in the air with that one small, noncommittal sentence. "You can take B12," he said. "I think. I might be wrong. It's one of the *B*s, I think." He instructed me to enter the search term into the search box on Google when I got home.

I didn't ask any more questions.

According to the Endometriosis Foundation of America, approximately one in ten people with female reproductive systems worldwide are diagnosed with endometriosis. Many of these people don't tell anyone about their symptoms because they're taught not to talk about them. An Australian study found that women feared breaching "menstrual etiquette" by talking about their symptoms; when they did discuss their symptoms, women were ostracized and belittled. And so, instead of speaking, we live inside of a story we don't quite understand, a story set in darkened bathrooms and bedrooms, a story with a plot that rises and falls inside what we've been told are the darkest parts of the human body. Because we've been taught that our stories, that the blood and fear and vomit and pain inside our stories, are unspeakable, some of us don't speak about them at all, even to our doctors.

These kinds of silences are not without consequence. A 2006 study showed that 86 percent of women with chronic pelvic pain are also affected by depression; depression was detected in 38 percent of the women in the study without pelvic pain.

65

My senior year of college, I signed up for a class called The Talking Cure. I expected the course to cover the theory that through talking about what was happening in our minds, we could stop some of the painful things that happened in our bodies.

I did not expect for the course to cover my own history, or to read stories that sounded so much like my own.

Freud's mentors, Jean-Martin Charcot and Josef Breuer, studied women who'd developed a disorder in which their psychological issues were made manifest in physical symptoms. Later, Freud himself would follow in their footsteps. The disorder wasn't anything new, really. Records of it stretched back to ancient Greece. It's widely assumed but not confirmed that Hippocrates, in whose name all the doctors I saw swore to "tread with care in matters of life and death," gave this disorder its name: hysteria, from the Greek ὑστέρα or *hystera*—meaning uterus.

From Elaine Showalter's *The Female Malady*, I learned that hysteria was originally seen as a thing that could go wrong only in female bodies. Later, this was found to be untrue, as hysteria also happened in male bodies—including, presumably, the body of the narrator of Rainer Maria Rilke's semi-autobiographical novel, *The Notebooks of Malte Laurids Brigge*, and perhaps of Rainer Maria Rilke himself. But the ancient Greeks believed a woman's uterus could become untethered and float around in her body, like a ghost, like an uncaged beast. It was this floating uterus, they assumed, that caused the symptoms of hysteria: A cough. A twitch. A seizure. A silence. An inability to correctly place one foot in front of the other. An inability to correctly place one's self and one's body in time or space.

Breuer and Freud and their colleagues, however, thought the ancient Greeks were wrong. Instead of the womb roaming through the body, untethered and uncaged, they assumed these symptoms were the result of thoughts and feelings that the woman's mind had suppressed. They were a human version of steam peeping out of a teakettle: a way to release stress, a cry for attention to what was boiling inside.

66

I MIXED AN EFFERVESCENT CODEINE TABLET INTO COLD water. I mixed Wild Turkey with Diet Coke. I mixed half a teaspoon of blond lightening powder with two teaspoons of blond developing crème. I'd spent all day with the pain I'd spent all week with, the pain I'd walked with, clenching my teeth. I'd had a period for six months straight and tried every pill and herb and prayer the doctors suggested. Black cohosh. Yarrow. Four Motrin at once. Primrose and Provera. Lupron shots, heating pads, raspberry-leaf tea. I'd traded white wine for whiskey, acetaminophen for hashish. I'd cut holes in my shirts and my jeans. I'd worn safety pins as earrings. I'd whittled my signature down by the letter. I'd become Em. I'd become E.

I poured more Wild Turkey into a cup. I added more lightening powder but not more lightening crème. I did not perform a strand test for damage, as instructed. Instead, I let the whiskey hide the very idea of damage from me. I'd planned to bleach four chunks of my hair, wrapped in the foil I'd bought for leftover curry. I'd wrapped my eighth before I heard Leia yell, "Dude, what is *up* with you?" She'd been knocking on my dorm room door for days, she said, but I couldn't hear over the Radiohead album we'd both listened to for weeks, over its car crash of horns and keyboards.

I handed her the bottle of Wild Turkey. She chugged. I chugged. My scalp sizzled to the tune of the music, now bell-sweet and silver, Thom Yorke's falsetto ringing: *Release me, release me.* I held up the Super Blonde box and pointed to my head.

"I'm waiting to see," I yelled, "if blondes really do have more fun."
Leia raised her eyebrows and pursed her lips and nodded.

When I woke the next afternoon, I couldn't remember. What had happened after the bleach and shampoo, after we left our private music for a club's thud and bass? I told my friends it must be right, what they say about blondes and fun. It must've been a night of more fun than a girl should remember, anyway.

67

In 1882, Jean-Martin Charcot began a neurology clinic at the Salpêtrière Hospital in Paris. A skilled neurologist, Charcot was the first doctor to fully describe multiple sclerosis and to identify plaques on the brain as its cause. He was most famous, however, for studying hysteria, that female malady. At first, he theorized that the disease had a physical cause, some inherited disorder of the nervous system that seemed to strike only female patients. Toward the end of his career, having found no physical cause, he decided instead that the cause was psychological, rooted not in the branching roots of the nervous system but in some trauma that, once buried in the mind, sprouted and stretched its limbs through a woman's body. Freud himself traveled to study at the Salpêtrière in 1885; he translated Charcot's lectures into German, and this work became the soil from which his theory of psychoanalysis grew.

The Salpêtrière itself had deep and shifting roots. The building had not always been a hospital. It was first a gunpowder factory, then an asylum for poor and disabled women. By the time of the French Revolution in 1789, the Salpêtrière was both a prison for prostitutes and an asylum for indigent women the world deemed mad. In their cells, prostitutes waited to be herded onto ships and shipped off to the New World and away from France.

During the September Massacres of 1792, a mob thrashed against the Salpêtrière's locks, axing down the doors to rooms where the

prostitutes slept, their skirts wrapped tight around their legs to protect them from the rats' teeth. Some of the women were asleep, or not
sleeping but waiting. They blinked against torchlight, fought against
the hands that shoved them into the night. Or maybe they were too
tired to fight. Or maybe they saw that with the hands came faces, and
with those faces eyes that flashed with fear and wine and thrill. They
would have known that this meant a particular kind of danger, one
with which they were familiar.

By the time Charcot established his neurology clinic, the
Salpêtrière floated atop a manicured lawn thick with imported flowers: perhaps flowering almond for hope, columbine for salvation. There
were scrolled iron beds and bleached linens, a great hall, scrubbed
public latrines. Charcot's patients were hysterics, women whose bodies bent them into Cs, who, mute through the day, screamed their
own secret languages into the dark.

There were cream-skinned girls with slacked jaws, their perfect
pointed chins bearded with foamed spit. Charcot let his patients loose
from their locked chambers and into the great hall, where he led them
to put on a show for financial supporters. He hypnotized them until
they followed his commands, until the symptoms of hysteria became
the steps in a dance Charcot choreographed. They'd lift their skirts
to their knees and point their toes, or else curtsy with a smile, or else
fist their hands, thrusting them low into air. He directed them to
pantomime scenes: right knee bowed to floor and head down, then
raised fingers counting invisible beads, or else a hand outstretched
to the imagined man who hands her a gift, a sweet she places on her
tongue, eyelids lowered with pleasure at the taste.

Perhaps Charcot saw himself as an artist. Perhaps he sometimes
woke from dreams surprised to find his hands absent of clay. A "*visuel*," a seer—that's how Charcot described himself to Freud, who
later praised his artistic temperament. Charcot draped his patients
in fabric and beads, pinned feathers in their hair. When they shook,

the fabric caught and released the light. When they slept, one could imagine he saw their faces as paintings, cheeks flushed with a wash of vermillion, eyes safe and calm behind ocher lids. He started charging for his lectures, for performances in which he hypnotized his female patients until their bodies contorted in the seizured throws of *grand hystérie*.

It seems clear to me that Charcot saw his patients as the materials from which he created great art. It also seems clear to me that they lived lives not much different from the prostitutes locked inside the Salpêtrière's cells during the French Revolution. When I imagine them, I imagine that they felt themselves floating on the hands of a mob as dangerous as the mob that stormed the Salpêtrière during the September Massacres, a sea rushing down the cobblestone streets. I imagine them hypnotized, forced below the waters of their own conscious minds. I imagine them drowning. I imagine their bodies forced into performance, legs kicking as if they'd pushed their way to the surface. I imagine their eyes unstaring, the selves behind those eyes gone.

68

I DIDN'T KNOW HIM WELL.

How many women's stories start that way?

I didn't know him well. He was older. He was, Leia and I surmised, somewhere between thirty and forty. I was nineteen. I wouldn't have met him had I not taken that playwriting class. Had I not worked so hard to get into the class, had I not visited the professor twice and said what I hoped were impressive things until he relented and allowed me to audit the class. This was the only way that I could take playwriting and keep the promise I made to my mother.

"Emily," she'd said on the two-day drive from Alabama to New York, "promise me this: you will *not* get up here in New York and start taking acting classes. You're here to learn. You're here to prepare yourself for a career, not to play around."

I mumbled, "Yes," and nodded before pushing the Play button on my Walkman, letting the *Hair* soundtrack block out the sound of our tires crunching miles and miles of asphalt. I told myself that since this (1) wasn't an acting class and (2) wasn't for credit, I hadn't broken my promise to my mother. This became one of the reasons I blamed myself: I had no business being in that class in the first place and so, I told myself, what did I expect?

I didn't know the man's name for weeks. I knew him instead by the blank zero on the top of his head, which shone red with cold as he ascended the metal stairs that iced with an almost performative ease. I stood on the top landing, smoking Camel Lights with one ungloved hand. We'd stand together sometimes, waiting for the rest of the class to clang and clamor up, still ringing from voice lessons. We talked about Leonard Cohen, how his voice seemed more beautiful for its ugliness, for the smoke and whiskey veneering each note. We talked about the plays we liked, the spotlights and darknesses, the witches warning Macbeth that no matter what, no act done is ever undone. We didn't talk about our families or the landscapes we watched through half-lidded windows as we flew home to them. We didn't talk about high school mascots or gymnasiums or the rooms we'd found ourselves entering and exiting in all the years before we stood together on that landing. And perhaps because there was nothing personal between us, I felt it was safe to agree to a date with him. He'd been asking for two months. I wanted to be polite.

I wore the faux-suede coat I'd found on clearance for fifteen dollars. As we walked to the movie theater, our breath made clouds opaque as smoke.

"This coat seemed warm enough back in Alabama," I said, half breathless, and later I'd point to this moment as a fault. As if by walking us into the personal I had walked us through the threshold of a door I might not at that moment have recognized but for which I was entirely to blame. He wrapped his scarf around my neck, pulling it tight then releasing it, laughing at the panic that, I know, popped into my eyes.

I don't remember what movie we saw. I do remember the darkness, the way his hand crept to my leg. To my thigh. To the inside of my thigh. No matter how many times I pushed it away. When he reached for my hand, I relented. We were in a theater full of people. I told myself I was safe.

After the theater emptied itself and it was just him and me and all the barely lit sidewalks we had to walk, I began to feel it. A sickness, somewhere in my stomach. We held hands. He waited until we were under a streetlight to kiss me. I tasted the sour of his tongue. I told myself to stop being afraid.

On the stoop in front of my dorm, I stood on my toes to reach his lips for a good-night kiss. He pushed against me. He pushed my mouth open with his tongue. He asked if he could come in. I felt the sickness again.

"I'm just really tired," I said. "I'm sorry." Did I even finish speaking before he had covered my mouth with his, before he grabbed a wad of hair and yanked it, then pushed the back of my head until my lips slammed against his, until my teeth cut into my lips? He stuck his tongue in my mouth and I couldn't breathe, so I pushed against his chest. I couldn't get free. I couldn't get free and I couldn't breathe and I pushed. It wasn't working. So I moved my mouth until I felt the top of his tongue with my teeth.

I bit.

"What the hell." He yanked my hair before he let me go and wiped his mouth with one hand. "What the hell," he said, but I was on the stoop and thanking him for the movie and thanking God that the door was unlocked, and then I was slipping out of his reach, lung-emptyingly grateful that by the time he looked up and tried to follow after me, I'd locked the door behind me.

I didn't cry until I'd closed and locked the door to my room. Until I was standing, shaking, away from his hands and his tongue. "What the hell." I stood and shook. I couldn't remember how to sit down.

Later, I told some friends the story. We sat in a circle on my dorm room floor, passing a bottle of vodka around. They listened, eyebrows raised in an unfamiliar way. They tilted their heads to the side.

"It doesn't sound like he was trying to do anything bad," one friend said.

"It sounds like he was trying to be romantic," another friend said.

"Maybe he was just doing what he thought he was supposed to do," a third friend said.

I looked across the circle to Leia. I tried to give her a significant look, a look that meant *I am significantly in need of your help.* She gingerly took a sip from the vodka bottle then wiped the lip of it with her sweatshirt. She didn't look at me.

"I just don't think you totally get how dating works yet." Leia's voice sounded strange, soft, and I couldn't tell if she was embarrassed by what she'd said or by how totally I did not get how dating works.

I sat. I nodded. I lit a cigarette. I told myself it was possible that this was true. I was a virgin who'd had her first kiss at eighteen. From the time I started puberty, I'd associated my reproductive parts only with pain. With the cold steel of every doctor's office I'd visited since I started my period. I assumed the way I felt about sex was just another symptom, an extension of this pain.

"I guess I should've just gone with it," I said. "I guess I didn't understand."

Leia held the bottle up to me. I shook my head and stubbed the cigarette against the ashtray, then left to take a shower. When I scrubbed my scalp with shampoo, I felt the base of my skull, the raw spot where he had pulled my hair.

I didn't understand.

69

WHEN SHE WAS FIRST ADMITTED, THE AVERAGE PATIENT AT the Salpêtrière would've been close to the same age as I was in fifth grade. Her symptoms would've started like mine: a sneeze or cough, or else a mouth that suddenly tongued only silence, or a mouth that opened to sound only after midnight. The change would have been slight but sudden, as stubborn as her body, focused suddenly on change, growing breasts and hips, hair in places she knew as blank.

She would've spent her childhood stepping over branches with her brothers, chasing rabbits that leapt away from her footsteps as if sprung by a winding key. She would've studied books with etchings of animals accompanied by their names—*lapin, chat, chien*. In the summers, she'd ride trains to the sea with her family, sleeping in compartments cloaked by indigo velvet. She'd focus on one tree to see how long she could keep it in her window's square; then, when it flashed from her peripheral vision, she'd choose another spruce, or a white stone, or a house with a mustache of linked flowers balanced above its red mouth of a door.

When the sun fell, the light bulb inside her compartment opened its eye. She'd try to catch as many words as she could in her brother's book before he flipped the page—*onion, girl, ocean, gull*. She'd try to measure the ground as it rolled itself away on the way to the summer cottage, to its linens that smelled of oak drawers and dried rosemary. There were wave-smooth pebbles to fill her hands full of shore. There were forests, dense, and the white backs of her brothers who always made their footsteps wider and longer when she begged them to stay close. When the squares of their bodies grew dim, she would close her eyes and follow the crisp snap of twigs beneath their feet, or else she would watch the needle pricks of light between trees, the path as thin as a thread beneath her feet.

70

MY LAST SEMESTER OF COLLEGE, A GYNECOLOGIST SUGGESTED another round of Lupron after a laparoscopic uterosacral nerve ablation (LUNA), an experimental procedure in which he would sever the ligaments that attached my uterus to the peritoneum, the membrane silking the purse of my abdomen.

"That's where the nerve pathways are," he said. "Disrupt the pathways and, hopefully, you disrupt some of the pain." The nerves could grow back, he explained, and when they did, the pain might be different. It might feel like a sucker punch. It might feel like a burn. It might not work at all. But there was a chance that the procedure might buy me enough time to finish graduate school and, more importantly, to try to get married and/or have a child.

"'Might' is the best I'm going to get, isn't it?" I asked.

The gynecologist did not answer.

Neither did my mother, who thought this was a bad idea. All I could think of was the three years ahead of me, the night classes and night library visits and all-night sessions copying what I needed to know from library books into carefully organized notebooks for my classes. All I could think of was this: "might" is good enough if it means relief long enough for me to get my MFA.

I signed the papers.

•

According to a 2017 *Kaiser Health News* article, by 1999, when I was a sophomore in college and on my fourth round of Lupron, the FDA had received adverse-event reports from 6,000 patients treated with the drug. Christina Jewett, the article's author, mentions that by 2017, the FDA couldn't locate their 1999 report. However, Jewett writes that a summary of the report in court documents shows that the FDA found "high prevalence rates for serious side effects." According to Lupron's own prescribing information, adverse reactions reported after the drug's approval include "convulsion, peripheral neuropathy, paralysis . . . serious liver injury . . . spinal fracture . . . decreased white blood count . . . tenosynovitis-like symptoms . . . hypotension, hypertension, deep vein thrombosis, pulmonary embolism, myocardial infarction, stroke, [and] transient ischemic attack."

According to a KTNV Las Vegas news report, by 2019, the FDA had received more than 25,000 reports of adverse events related to the use of Lupron. This included more than 1,500 reports of deaths.

71

ACCORDING TO THE CURRENT PRESCRIBING INFORMATION on the Lupron Depot website, the span of a patient's first course of Lupron Depot should be no longer than six months. During this initial course of treatment, the patient may or may not take five milligrams of norethindrone acetate—progesterone—as an add-back therapy to mitigate certain side effects. If the patient's first course of Lupron Depot is unsuccessful, the patient can receive another six months of treatment with the drug. This second round must be accompanied by add-back therapy. However, according to the website, no patient should undergo treatment with Lupron Depot, with or without add-back therapy, for longer than a total of twelve months. Notably, the prescribing information states that the postapproval adverse reactions occurred *with* the use of add-back therapy.

Between the ages of eighteen and twenty-two, I kept an almost-daily diary. The doctors and insurance company also kept insisting that I try Lupron again, and so I kept trying Lupron again. When I was not treated with Lupron, I was treated with Depo-Provera, a contraceptive injection used to treat endometriosis, or other oral contraceptives. Though the diary is heavily redacted with Sharpie markers and scissors, there remain at least 172 references to wanting to die, praying that I would die, and/or a preference to die rather than continue to live inside of my body with the symptoms that the medications either did not adequately treat or caused.

Still, I wonder sometimes how much worse it would've been without these treatments. I wonder a lot of the time how much worse it must be for people who don't have access to medications or treatments.

I destroyed most of my diaries with Sharpie markers and scissors because I was afraid. I was afraid that one day I'd no longer be able to take it, the blood and the blood and the pain. I didn't want my parents to know how long I'd wanted it all to end. I wanted them, just in case, to think it was an accident. I didn't want, just in case, for them to remember all the papers they'd signed. I didn't want them to take on blame.

By the time I turned thirty, it was clear: all my stalling tactics had failed. The nerves threading my uterus to my peritoneum had grown back, and in place of the cramps I once had came a terrible burning, as if the inside of my abdomen flamed with an actual, inextinguishable fire. I canceled a lot of plans. I ran out of excuses. I was in the middle of winter in the middle of a three-year visiting assistant professorship at a small college in Kentucky, and no matter how cold it got, my body felt like fire.

I finally told my best friend, Deena, "I'm sorry, I'm getting my period and it feels like I'm burning."

"Burning?" she asked.

"Like actual fire."

"You do realize that's not normal, right?"

I nodded into the phone and then realized she couldn't see, and so I said yes.

Thirty minutes later, Deena showed up at my front door. She'd driven through the winter's first snow over the twisted back roads between her apartment and mine. She handed me a bottle of bourbon.

"Don't you dare change out of your pajamas," she said, already walking toward the kitchen cabinet where I kept my shot glasses. We filled the glasses to the brim before clinking them against each other, raising our eyebrows and saying, "Cheers," with a solemn gravity.

Later, I pulled snow boots over my pajama pants and zipped myself into my puffiest coat. "I feel like a marshmallow," I said, shoving my hands in my pockets to search for the gloves I kept in them.

"There's a reason for that," Deena said. She opened the front door and gestured for me to walk outside. We struggled our way to the right side of my apartment, where the complex ended and a tangled field stretched out like a mess of unkempt green hair. We bent down and grabbed handfuls of snow, packing them into tight balls before facing the brick side of my apartment, letting our boots slide into the snow, testing our footing for traction.

Deena nodded in my direction. "Do it," she said. "Show that fucker how you feel."

I took a deep breath. I knew and didn't know that it was cold. I knew and didn't know that was because I was drunk. I lifted the snowball high over my head and threw it as hard as I could, and as it shattered against the brick, I could not help but scream.

72

As a girl who'd later become a patient at the Salpêtrière grew older, before the blood and the pain, before her body had fully taken the shape others would identify as a woman's, before her body took control and twisted itself into movements she neither willed nor understood, she learned new ways to button her body in dresses, her feet into leather ankle boots. She plaited her hair with ribbons, sucked in her breath as her mother tightened her corset. She stood in front of the mirror and failed to recognize herself, her body, the shape it was growing into: not the solid square of her brothers but a curve like the sand timer her mother used to soft-boil eggs.

The morning she began to bleed, she woke to the thought of chickens plucked down to their skins, or of valises filled with silk dressing gowns, or of the curls that fell down her mother's back once released from pins and hat. She thought of the pearl inlaid in the etched silver of her mother's hand mirror, the needle's glint between two fingers as it pierced stretched klostern with embroidery thread. She thought of how much it hurt when her mother pulled her hair tight, the smear of red her dancing shoes painted between her two longest toes. The morning she began to bleed, there was no warning nor explanation.

Her mother shushed her, splashed water on her hot face, then gave her a washcloth soaked in water and perfume. There were bundles of rags, a hush in the hallway, a mattress. The sheets reached up to her chin. There were tonics that reeked of liquor and lime, handkerchiefs soaked in vinegar, in wine. There were her brothers' valises

packed with white shirts, play trousers, and then the train that took
her brothers away while she stood on the platform, trying to keep
sight of their faces, their windows, until they were motion, until they
vanished for the summer, leaving her and her mother behind.

She felt the strange voice in her throat. All through the night
it bled out of her. Then the voice decided that it liked day as well,
and she listened, patient, curious, as it pushed through the garden
walk, as it shrieked into the pail of cow's milk. Her mother called
the doctor, and according to his instructions, she was stripped. Her
limbs fought against the bathtub full of ice. Her hands wanted to be
claws. Her feet rose and shattered the water. The doctor held her under until her hands dyed themselves blue. Still, her voice roamed the
house and its hallways. Her voice filled her brothers' beds, turned the
pages of schoolbooks locked far from her reach. Then the men came
with their cold instruments. They measured her chest's thud and fall.
They palmed her knees apart. They soaked rags red with her blood,
led leeches from glass jars to the raw spot between her legs that she
tried to vise shut. Still, her voice remained the bad patient who would
never behave, until the doctors told her parents: if she remained in the
house, the family would have no peace. But there was somewhere for
her to go, a hospital, a good one. Her parents paid the doctors, and
they took her and her body and its strangeness away.

73

Two days after my seventh laparoscopy, my right leg just didn't feel right. This is because my right leg just did not feel. Period. My enormous cat clambered over it, and though I knew her paws needled the skin, I didn't feel it.

"Okay," I said out loud to my leg. "That's weird." I poked the place where my cat's paws and claws had been. Nothing. I pinched the place I'd poked. Nothing. I lifted my arm up in a right angle to my body and turned the hand at the end of that arm into a fist. I let that fist fall, hard, on the place on my leg.

Nothing.

The gynecologist and his nurses were at first receptive. "That is totally normal," his nurses said after consulting him. "It happens all the time. It's just because of the position we have to put you in for surgery. Sometimes a nerve will get pinched and you'll feel numb for a while, but the feeling will come back sooner or later."

I waited. Sooner, the feeling did not come back. Later, the feeling did not come back. Instead, the non-feeling spread from a small numb circle on my right thigh to a large numb circle on my right thigh. Then the nonfeeling spread outside of a circle and to my entire thigh. Sooner or later, the gynecologist and his nurses still assured me, the nonfeeling would begin to feel.

The nonfeeling did not begin to feel, sooner or later.

I did begin to feel something, and sooner: my pelvic pain, which came again in crashing, crushing kinds of waves. During what would be my last appointment with him, I told the gynecologist that my nonfeeling leg still didn't feel, but I had begun to feel pain in my abdomen. The gynecologist did not look at me. The gynecologist tapped his pen against my file.

"Well, there's only one option left," he said, "and that's Lupron."

I looked at him. I looked at him not looking at me. His pen was capped. He was not writing anything down, and he was not planning to.

"But we talked about that," I said. The gynecologist's left eyebrow left its spot and arched just enough to make a point.

"With endometriosis this aggressive, that's the only course of treatment left."

"But I've tried that before. I tried for years." I could hear tears choking my voice, which made me feel desperate and angry but mostly embarrassed. "I can't do it again. I'm sorry. I just can't do it again."

The gynecologist looked at me. He had blue eyes, I realized, and they were cold blue, stone blue, the kind of blue that writers call piercing, the kind of blue that writers place in the faces of villains who are sharply incapable of sympathy. His eyebrow arched and his lips did, too, as if this were a moment he wanted to enjoy. "Are you refusing this treatment?"

I looked at him. He looked at me. We both knew what this meant. "I am."

My time as his patient was over.

I didn't cry as I put my clothes back on, as I waited in line at the checkout counter, as I gave the receptionist my credit card and signed my receipt with her pen, which was covered in green florist's tape and had a fabric daisy on the top. I didn't cry until I was in the hallway waiting for the elevator, and I didn't stop crying when a man stepped into the women's center elevator with me, awkwardly carrying a bouquet of carnations and a copy of the *Lexington Herald-Leader*.

•

Four months later, on October 20, 2010, the FDA's Division of Drug Marketing, Advertising, and Communications sent a letter to Sanofi-Aventis, the then-makers of Lupron, notifying them of "the need to add new safety information to the Warnings and Precautions section of the drug labels." In the letter, the FDA declared that Sanofi-Aventis's promotional materials were misleading because they omitted many of the possible consequences of Lupron. These include increases in a patient's risk of diabetes and of cardiovascular problems, including stroke and heart attack. The letter also warns that patients may experience spinal cord compression, which could lead to paralysis and other complications—some of which may be fatal.

When the doctor suggested that round of Lupron, he didn't inform me of any of the FDA's recent tests, warnings, suggestions, revisions, and notifications.

There was no reason for him to inform me. I was a female patient.

All of the FDA's tests, warnings, suggestions, revisions, and notifications related to the use of Lupron in male patients and male patients only.

In their May 2010 news release, the FDA did acknowledge that "some GnRH agonists are also used in women," however, they didn't say if female patients faced the same risks as male patients. That wasn't because GnRH agonists don't cause problems for female patients. It was because neither the FDA nor the pharmaceutical companies knew if GnRH agonists caused problems for female patients. No one had tried to find out. "There are no known comparable epidemiologic studies evaluating the risk of diabetes and cardiovascular disease in women taking GnRH agonists," the FDA stated.

74

In order for a doctor to perform pelvic surgery, the nurses arrange the patient's body in a position that resembles the position in which nurses arrange a woman's body during childbirth. The position has a name—the lithotomy position—and it looks, approximately, like a cartoon lightning bolt lying on its side. The patient lies on the operating table, her head near the top, her bottom positioned just against the bottom edge of the table. The patient's legs are lifted so that the knees are approximately above the tips of her hip bones. The calves rest in stirrups, which are held up by metal bars. The feet dangle up in the air, useless and flimsy as decorative tassels.

The lithotomy position makes things easier for the physician. It can make things much harder for the patient. When it comes to childbirth, for instance, the position allows the physician to tend to the patient easily, but it also narrows the birth canal, making delivery far from easy. An article in *The Journal of Minimally Invasive Gynecology* also notes that when a patient is not positioned correctly in the lithotomy position, the patient is at risk of injury "to lower extremity nerves, including the femoral, lateral femoral cutaneous, obturator, sciatic, and common peroneal nerves." A 2000 study found that keeping patients in the lithotomy position for over two hours "was strongly associated with [lower extremity] neuropathies."

•

Before another doctor performed my eighth laparoscopy, we had a difficult appointment. It did and did not seem difficult at the time. It involved a conversation that had happened so many times it felt more like a routine, just one more test that the doctors found necessary.

The difficult conversation begins like this: I tell the physician that even after surgery and hormonal treatments, I am experiencing pelvic and vaginal pain, especially around the time of my periods, which come twice a month.

The physician responds by informing me that I cannot be experiencing pelvic and vaginal pain, and that though it might seem like I'm having periods, it's just breakthrough bleeding caused by birth control pills, even if I have to wear a tampon with an overnight pad.

"Birth control pills," the physician informs me, "have been shown to stop the growth of endometriosis." Since I was taking a medication that has been shown to stop the growth of endometriosis, it follows, my endometriosis must not have been growing, which means that I must not actually have experienced pelvic and vaginal pain.

"But I am," I inform the physician. "I am experiencing pain. Sometimes it gets so bad that I can hardly move. I throw up. I pass out. I can't take it," I say, and as soon as I say, "I can't take it," I know that I have made a mistake. I know what is coming.

"Ah," the physician will respond, because my words have opened a door that the physician will walk through, and fast.

And this is exactly what the gynecologist did in that difficult appointment. He told me that he'd seen this before, this kind of pelvic and vaginal pain, which, he said, is a sexual problem.

"This kind of sexual problem," he said, "is very common in women who were molested as children."

"But I wasn't molested as a child," I said.

He was not listening. "All the psychological trauma related to your molestation manifests itself in pelvic and vaginal pain, and in a lack of sexual arousal."

"But I wasn't molested, and I'm not talking about sexual arousal," I said.

He was still not listening.

He was, instead, still talking, without even taking a not-quite pause: "The pain may feel physical, but it's entirely mental. It's all a trick of the mind."

"So you're saying that I'm imagining things."

He paused long enough to give me a look that was significant mainly due to its condescension. "I'm saying that the pain can *feel* very real. I'm saying that pelvic and vaginal pain is a common response to sexual abuse experienced in early childhood."

"Except that I didn't experience sexual abuse in early childhood because I was not molested as a child." As I spoke, I realized that I was crying. I realized that I couldn't stop the crying. I realized that I was confused. I was in so much pain and I was so tired. Had I experienced sexual abuse? Was that the thing that happened with my fifth-grade teacher, the thing that placed a cough in my throat and kept it there for two weeks, so that I wouldn't have to go to school? I was in so much pain. I was so tired. "Okay." I heard a voice that sounded like mine, but it was too distant for me to control. "I had this teacher, when I was a kid. She was—strange. It was a strange situation. It wasn't abuse like that, though. Nothing like that happened. I was not molested. But it was just strange."

After I gave him my confession, he gave me another significant look. He gave me the name and number of a psychotherapist who specialized in sexual trauma. He gave me the name and number of the assistant who scheduled surgeries for him. He gave me my folder and told me to follow the blue arrows to the checkout desk.

I drove home. I asked myself: *Am I crazy?*

I asked myself: *Is it all in my head, all this pain? And how can it be all in my head if there is also so much blood?*

I asked myself: *What was I supposed to say?*

I didn't answer. I cried. And the landscape of highways and cars and red lights and green lights smeared across my field of vision. It didn't answer either.

I was so tired.

75

THE WOMEN OF CHARCOT'S SALPÊTRIÈRE WEREN'T CHAINED to bed frames. They weren't tied into straightjackets they couldn't untie. They weren't hidden behind doors with double locks and windows only wide enough for wardens to make sure they stayed sedated. They were, instead, forced to perform and in a way that made them famous: Blanche Wittman, "Queen of the Hysterics." Louise Augustine Gleizes, who for five years sat in a trance for photographs, or allowed her body to dance wild for a gray-suited crowd. Charcot led his patients into a lecture hall packed with people who wore Paris's most expensive clothes, then arranged the women upon a stage. He hypnotized the women whose bodies held the most talent, using a pocket watch to coax them into sleep while standing still. While their minds were elsewhere, unaware, their bodies became his. Perhaps they dreamed of lovers in rooms lacking light. Perhaps they thought of his fingers' warmth. Perhaps they did not think at all. Perhaps they knew that this wasn't a way out, but that it might be a way up, at least.

He pressed a hand to their cheeks and their lips went slack. Then their lips drew back together, wet with foamed spit he'd thumb away before the audience could see. Their pasts curled into the present and unfurled, shaping their bodies into the same patterns again and again and again.

The back curved down, parietal bone nearing the floor. The hands given to the air and twisted. The leg turned until its heel faced the stage's apron. Last, the act that packed them in daily, the contortions that Charcot named *attitudes passionnelles*: a woman lying on a bare wood stage, left hand stroking the side of her face, which moved to meet it as her hips began to shift, slow, a rhythm from right to left to match the rhythm of Charcot's watch, the rhythm of the whole room leaning and breathing. Back lifted and curved, breasts rising in two curves and then falling again, her hips lifted from the stage floor as the audience lifted their own bodies from their seats, coughed into hands cupped to half-cover their eyes. At last she screamed a sound that filled a space between release and terror, until she slid limp to the stage, slack and empty, staring at a ceiling she did not see, or at the audience, who had seen what she would never see, the confession she never willed herself to perform.

I always forgot the rules of confession as soon as I stepped into that cubicle and looked into the darkness of the screen. I knew that Father Frank hid like God behind it, and I knew that he was about to be very disappointed in me and my sins, if he wasn't already. From what I had learned in catechism class, I knew that the punishments my body meted out had to be justified by what I had done and what I had failed to do. And so I would forget the rules. I'd forget when to cross myself—before or after kneeling? I'd forget if I needed to kneel in the first place, or if I recited the Act of Contrition before or after I recited the list of sins I'd been collecting every afternoon after school, like sharp, painful stones. Sometimes I would say, "I am hardily sorry for my sins," instead of, "I am heartily sorry for my sins." Sometimes I would say, "I am hardly sorry for my sins." I'd wonder, later, if this was why I never felt forgiven.

76

MY MOTHER HAD ONE FEAR: THAT I'D BE WHEELED INTO AN operating room and I wouldn't come back alive.

She and my father sat in the waiting room through seven surgeries. Each time, the doctor emerged, serious and in scrubs, to show them the photographs he'd taken during the procedure. Each time, they knew that I was okay because the doctor spoke to them in the waiting room. Had anything gone wrong, they'd be moved into a little room for privacy instead.

On the day of my eighth surgery, my mother was alone. My father had planned to drive from the Alabama dealership where he worked as an accountant to my Kentucky hospital as soon as he closed out for the month. By this point, my laparoscopies were routine: the waiting room became the presurgical holding area became the surgical theater became the recovery room became the (hopefully) private room in which my parents and the doctors and I waited for me to be able to pee on my own, at which point I'd be released and wheeled to my parents' car. We were all so comfortable with the way things were supposed to happen. I told my father to stay, to close out. I told my father I'd see him when I got back to my apartment, at the point with pain pills where I'd say entertaining things. So my mother was alone when, about thirty minutes after I'd been taken back to the operating room, she watched a nurse scan the waiting room before asking for the Bolden family. My mother raised her hand and felt her heart thud, thud, a sound echoed by the nurse's fast footsteps.

"Is he finished already?" my mother asked.

"Oh no," the nurse said. The nurse was shaking. My mother could tell she was angry. And when the nurse told her to follow her to the little room, my mother knew exactly where this was going. But my mother knew she had to be strong. My mother was not crying. My mother made herself calm.

I woke from surgery into white. Unfeeling, fuzzed over. I saw only white, white, white.

There was a large plastic tube in my right nostril. This was unpleasant and unexpected. I tried to touch my nose and the tube inside of it. An alarm went off. I was very sleepy. Faces ballooned around my bed. Someone held down my arms and someone told me to stay still. There had been an accident, the balloons told me. A puncture. My small bowel. I'd be okay, but I needed to be very, very still. Then there was a hand, and then the hand injected something into the IV strung to my arm. I was very sleepy. A thought floated up through the white.

"Do I have a colostomy bag?" I asked.

"No," the balloons said, "no, no, you don't," and then they disappeared and took the recovery room with them.

77

My mother is the person everyone calls during an emergency. Stomach flu, surgery, death, divorce, injury—my mother is the person everyone calls. When one of my cousins had a brain tumor removed, my mother sat in her hospital room, reading a romance novel while my cousin slept, handing her iced ginger ales and making sure the straw pointed toward her lips first, holding her up by the armpits and walking her to the bathroom. They took the tumor out through her sinus cavity and then her nose, and then they packed her nostrils with cotton. When the time came to remove the packing, my aunt left to get a cup of coffee. She didn't come back, at least not in time for them to take the batting out.

My mother stayed.

My mother sat on the bed with my cousin, holding both of her hands. "They have to do this," my mother said, "so you have to be strong and let them."

Of course my cousin cried. Of course my cousin shook. Of course my cousin knew the kind of pain she was about to experience. Of course my mother did, too, and of course my mother knew that she'd been left with the responsibility of carrying her through this pain, which also meant the responsibility of carrying the experience of watching her, teenaged and tiny, shaking as the doctors pulled out the bloody cotton packed in her nose.

Of course my mother stayed.

And without being there, I can still visualize if not the pain my cousin experienced then what my mother experienced, how she made herself strong so that my cousin could be strong, how she seemed unbreakable, untouchable, every wrinkle of worry or fear smoothed out in the expression she made when she told you to be strong. The green glitter of her eyes, widened. The tone of voice sharpened into the same tone she used when reprimanding you because she knew it was the only way you'd pay attention, the only way you'd square your shoulders and sink your teeth against one another and do what you damn well had to do because the doctors demanded it. Without being there, I can still imagine her, stern and strong and straight-backed, pulling my cousin into a hug and patting her back until her mother came back, until my mother gathered her purse and her romance novel and her just-in-case sweater, until my mother's heels tapped the hospital hallway's tile in a brisk and orderly pattern, until she walked into the parking lot and hit the Unlock button on her key fob, until she heard the answering beep that told her where she'd parked her car, until she opened the door and put her purse and her romance novel and her just-in-case sweater in the passenger seat, until she carefully locked the doors and checked to make sure no one could see in before folding her body over the steering wheel and letting it loose, a guttural, gut-shaking sob.

78

This is how my surgical accident happened.

Before I agreed to an operation, the surgeon performed a diagnostic ultrasound to see how things looked inside of my body.

Things did not look particularly good inside of my body.

Things looked particularly not good inside of my body because adhesions had rubber-roped my large and small intestines together, then tied them to places where they didn't belong. For this reason, the surgeon decided to insert the laparoscope through a small incision above my pubic bone rather than through a small incision in my navel in the hopes of avoiding the bowel.

This was not a good decision.

As the laparoscope went inside of my body, it did the very thing the surgeon was trying to avoid. It punctured my small bowel. This was a sort-of funny kind of thing, if not a ha-ha funny kind of thing, and it's why there was a plastic tube in my right nostril. The tube went all the way into my stomach, where it sucked out a green liquid and deposited it into a receptacle.

It was important to suck out the green liquid because my digestive system had to be shut down.

It was important to shut down my digestive system because, by piercing my small intestine, the surgeon had put me at risk for sepsis, which is, according to Healthpages.wiki, "a potentially fatal whole-body inflammation (a systemic inflammatory response syndrome or SIRS) caused by severe infection."

It was important for me to look up the definition on my phone right there, in my hospital bed, because the doctor never explained exactly why my body was in so much danger that he had to stick a tube down my nose.

Even under the morphine, the irony did not escape me: I spent much of my time in the classroom explaining to my students why they shouldn't use a wiki as a reliable source, yet here I was, in the hospital, asking a wiki about what was happening to my body because it seemed a far more reliable source than my own doctor.

Because it was the Memorial Day weekend, the hospital was understaffed, so they'd taken me to the cardiac floor. After my mother told him about the accident, my father drove to Kentucky and came straight to my hospital room. He kissed me on the forehead and said, "Hey, kid," in a voice so strained I knew he was trying, and hard, not to cry. My mother didn't even ask how fast he'd been going, to make it to Kentucky so soon. I spent most of my time itching from morphine and sleepless from the endless beeping of heart monitors. Three times a day, I walked the floor's circle with one of my parents, slowly, to avoid blood clots and build my strength. Through the opened doors I saw the other patients, gray shadows in shadowed gray beds. I wondered if they were ghosts. I wondered if I was.

Every few hours, a nurse came into my room. They emptied the receptacle of its green liquid and smiled patiently while I tried to tell a joke. The jokes went like this: "Well, I've been saying I need to go on a diet" and "I wanted to lose weight, but this is a little extreme" and "Is that Nickelodeon slime?" Sometimes the jokes got a ha-ha response, which made me feel satisfied, even if the nurses were only ha-haing because they knew I might be dying.

"You've told that joke four times," my mother said.

"It's a good one," I said. "I'm sure I'll tell it again." My mother sighed and looked down at her romance novel, shaking her head.

•

It is possible that I was, in fact, dying. The surgeon had neglected to (1) suggest or administer a full bowel-prep prior to surgery or (2) suggest or administer intravenous antibiotics into my body prior to surgery. This meant that whatever had been in my small intestine—acid, bacteria, bile—before surgery was still in my small intestine during surgery. And whatever had been in my small intestine during surgery seeped into my abdomen, where there were no antibiotics to fight off possible infection while my body waited to be repaired.

And my body had to wait quite a long time. My mother doesn't know how much time, exactly.

"Don't give a specific number," she tells me when I ask. "You don't have all the records for that surgery, and I don't want anyone to come back at you." I hear the fear edging into her voice, a fear with which I'm very familiar. Because it has its weight. Every time a doctor questions what you say, what you experience, what you know, marrow-deep, of your own body. It has its weight, and that weight is fear. It is difficult to trust in your experience of the body when the people you trust to take care of that body deny that your experience is true. And so we do not like to talk about the particulars, my mother and I, without the data to back it up. We do not like to talk about the particulars until they are there, typeset and time-stamped, in the doctor's own words: *here is the moment he picked up the scalpel, here the incision, here, right here, the mistake that was the doctor's, not mine.* I keep my silence, which is, after all, the only thing so many doctors wanted from me.

These are the particulars I do know.

The gynecological surgeon either (1) could not or (2) would not perform the small bowel repair. Instead, he called in a general surgeon who either (1) agreed to, as a favor, or (2) was forced to perform the small bowel repair.

The general surgeon was not in the hospital.

The general surgeon was with his daughter in a movie theater. The general surgeon was theoretically on call, but he didn't expect to actually receive a call. Only routine procedures (such as abdominal laparoscopies) that typically do not end in fatal or near-fatal accidents (such as bowel punctures) were scheduled on holiday weekends.

The general surgeon (1) left the movie theater, (2) drove to the hospital, and (3) prepared his body to perform a surgical procedure. He thoroughly scrubbed his hands and arms with antiseptic soap. He changed into sterile garments specifically designed for surgery, including a mask, a full-body suit, special shoes, and gloves.

This took quite a bit of time.

And during that quite-a-bit-of-time, my whole-body lay on a table in the operating room, abdomen open, insides exposed. The surgical team tried to keep the inside and outside of my body sterile. They tried to prevent the fluids leaking out of my intestines from entering my abdomen. But my body had to wait so long. Even after the small bowel had been repaired, they weren't sure what fluids leaked or where, and so my digestive system had to be shut down for four days. Were I to eat or drink or otherwise use my digestive system, my whole-body would be even more at risk, even closer to not-being.

79

As Charcot's fame grew, he threw the women—or rather, their watchers—public balls. At *Le Bal des folles*, the women who, onstage, shimmied shoulders beneath feathered headdresses, whose ankles sang with their bells as Charcot played them, now demurred, hid their faces behind fans, twisted hand in hand at their waists. They knew to watch a pocket for gold's glint. They knew that the handkerchief dotted with a wife's perfume hid fifty-franc coins that a man would press into their hands.

In the hospital, Charcot taught them how to act like women who held a secret even from themselves, who swallowed like a lozenge the last vestige of whatever memory led them to the hospital, the stage, the ballroom with heads lowered and wreathed in curls. They never whispered of escape. They never pressed too close against the men who paid to dance with a madwoman. They never leaned into the groomed hair stuck by pomade to his ear to say the words they screamed in trances, from under the writhing tide of *grande hystérie*: *bâtard, bâtard*, or else *laissez-moi être libre*.

80

FOR FOUR DAYS, I ATE ONLY CRUSHED ICE, METERED OUT three small spheres at a time. I sipped water and sucked on wet sponges. Then it was time to remove my nasal gastric tube. Finally. And I was terrified. I remember the expectation of pain. My mother held my hand and told me to look at her, not the nurses or the end of my nose or the tube inside of it. Her face, resolute, settled into a stern approximation of bravery that nevertheless betrayed the fact that she didn't want to see her daughter going through this. I wondered how many times she'd sat on the edge of my bed like this, smoothing back my hair and putting wet washrags on the back of my neck, placing a trash can in front of me at the precise angle necessary to catch whatever came out of the body that always seemed to betray me, which felt, by extension, like I was betraying her. She would never say I owed her, but I felt like I did. So I looked at her. I saw her face, resolute. I tried it on, or tried to: an expression set sternly into an approximation of bravery.

"Okay, just breathe in," the nurse said.

I looked at my mother.

"Take a deep breath," the nurse said.

I looked at my mother. I took a deep breath. The nurse leaned over. I saw the edge of her hand at the edge of my peripheral vision. My mother squeezed my hand, just a little, just gently. I kept looking at her.

"Now breathe out, slowly," the nurse said, extending the word *slowly* as if trying to convince me that words themselves were nothing but breath. I looked at my mother. Her nostrils flared in a way that suggested she too was taking a deep breath then letting it out slowly. I did the same. I wanted so desperately to be good. I wanted her to at least be able to see me doing this one good thing. I focused so intently on wanting to be good that I almost didn't notice the pain. I almost didn't notice the sickening slide of the tube coming out through my nose—"You're doing so good," my mother said, "just hang on, you're doing so good"—and then it was out.

There was nothing.

Just a strange feeling, an odd small awareness, as if I now recognized my body as a place where things had been but now were not. A private place where trespassers had entered and then left. My mother nodded and I nodded back to her. I tried to smile. I tried to mean it, to make it mean that I was going to be okay.

I hadn't slept in two days. The morphine kept me itching and awake. The nurse who had pulled out and repositioned the tube changed my morphine to Dilaudid. She told my parents to head back to my apartment, to get some sleep and take hot showers. "Don't worry," she said. "She'll be out like a light in a few minutes."

After my parents left, she taught me how to follow the hands on the clock as they traced a new path to the time when I could hit the button for more pain medication. "You're going to get some rest now," she said. "I am damn well going to make sure you're not in pain." She turned on the television and flipped through the channels until she found a *Bridezillas* marathon.

"That is my favorite," I told her, half asleep.

"I know," she said. "Let yourself go to sleep." I nodded and watched her as she walked out, and then I went to sleep.

81

In 1731, the Virgin Mary appeared to Saint Alphonsus Liguori as a young girl veiled in white. He later wrote a bedroom prayer through which one offers the hours of one's sleep to Jesus Christ one's God. Liguori's prayer also includes a request for Jesus Christ one's God to protect the sleeper during their hours of sleep, which implies that one can sin during one's sleep, that one can sin without even intending to sin, just as one can dream without even intending to dream.

When I attended Catholic school, I learned a lot about sins and the ways that God punishes us for them. I learned that if something very bad happens to you, it happens for a reason. I learned that that reason is you.

When my mother and the gynecologist spoke in that little room, the gynecologist had only just made the initial incision. He hadn't gotten much further than that when he realized he had punctured my bowel. He held up his hands. He stopped operating. My pelvis flooded with whatever had been in my bowel: acid, bacteria, bile. He couldn't have seen anything. But when he went to speak with my mother, alone, in that little room, he changed the facts of that sentence. Instead of "I couldn't see anything," he told her there was nothing to see. He told her that I had no endometriosis, that there was no physical evidence of any physical cause for my pain.

"It is my opinion," he told my mother, "that the pain is not in Emily's body. It is my opinion that the pain is in Emily's head."

My mother didn't know what to think. My mother didn't know what to say, and so she didn't say anything for a while. She listened to the clock. She doesn't remember how many times it ticked. "I thought you said you punctured her bowel with the first incision," she said, finally.

"I did," the gynecologist said. It was a statement that required a great deal of explanation, specifically in terms of how he knew I had no endometriosis if he hadn't had even begun to look for endometriosis. He did not choose to explain. Instead, while I lay open and prone in my body on the operating table, while the nurses suctioned and swabbed and sucked out the fluids flowing out of my small intestine, he chose to tell my mother that the origin of my pain was not endometriosis but sexual abuse.

"Sexual abuse?" My mother sat for a minute, the room whirling around her, while the gynecologist looked at her in a peculiar kind of way, somewhere between absolute terror and complete condescension. "Wait a minute," she said. "Her teacher?"

The gynecologist, she says, looked startled. He tipped his head backward, chin tipped upward. "Oh," he said. "I didn't think she had told you about him."

"She told me about *her*," my mother said, and I know her voice was high and loud. I know her right hand rose to her face, and I know that she moved it to the side, like she was waving off a wasp. "It was a woman. Nothing sexual happened. She got over that years ago."

The gynecologist sat for a moment, blinking, head still tilted backward. "Oh," he said, then "Oh," again. They sat for a moment. The clock ticked. "Well. She also has a sizable fibroid."

My mother nodded, kept her silence.

It has its weight. Every single time.

82

AFTER THE SUCCESS OF HIS LECTURE HALL, CHARCOT BUILT an atelier—an artist's studio—in quarters where prisoners once scratched at the rat bites on their ankles. He hired Albert Londe as a full-time photographer. Charcot developed a treatment based on the work of Luigi Galvani, the Bolognese physician who noticed a dead frog's leg kicked to life when static electricity traveled through a scalpel to spark its sciatic nerve. He saw the nerves and spine as a map of the body's dim lights, signaling motion and rest through flesh by flashing to bright then fading. Charcot tried Galvani's work on frogs on the human body: specifically, the bodies of his most stubborn patients, the women who stayed still onstage and in Albert Londe's atelier, immune to hypnosis. Charcot slipped electrodes, sharp as needles, under their skin to shock their muscles into movement. In that way, in front of Londe's camera, he moved those whose limbs he could not otherwise convince to perform.

The shutter opens: Mlle Bairet, black-clad and brass-buttoned, sits sleeping in a straight-backed chair as Charcot presses a slim baton against her nerves, using faradic shocks to bend her elbows in *V*s and bring them down again. The shutter closes. In Londe's four photographs, she could be in conversation, or else in a pause used to wave a mistaken phrase away. She could be telling a story about bad luck to a friend over a lunch of bread and salted tomatoes. She could be searching for the word she never remembers: the color of a fox's fur, the fleshy pads of their feet.

At the Salpêtrière, Londe developed a four-lensed camera to catch each twitch and jump of the *grande hystérie*. He later used his inventions to photograph men's muscles straining in play, how their eyes lifted and shifted. He took portraits of clowns, grins painted wide over their unsmiling mouths. He took photos of a criminal examined after death, head snapped back, torso a bloated oval. Not even a flap of skin remains to cover the neck, slit and peeled to see what lay inside—crude muscle, dried vein—and how it once made a voice.

83

I THOUGHT I KNEW ONE CERTAIN THING ABOUT THE Hippocratic oath: that in order for doctors to become doctors, they had to swear that they would first do no harm.

That one certain thing is completely and utterly wrong.

In order to become a doctor, a person instead swears to this: "I will follow that system of regimen which, according to my ability and judgement, I consider for the benefit of my patients, and abstain from whatever is deleterious and mischievous."

In the Latin translation of the original Greek oath, the final phrase reads: "*noxamvero et maleficium propulsabo.*" While *maleficium* does translate as "mischief," it also translates as "witchcraft": the word used in the European witch trials to describe the actions of *maleficae*, or witches. The word appears, most notably, in the *Malleus Maleficarum*—the handbook for identifying, trying, and killing witches used by the inquisitors in early modern Europe.

It goes without saying. These witches were women.

In October 2001, TAP Pharmaceutical Products, the joint venture of Abbott Laboratories and Takeda Chemical Industries that manufactured and marketed Lupron, received a number of criminal and civil charges.

One charge: TAP Pharmaceutical Products allegedly committed health-care fraud via Medicaid and Medicare.

Another charge: TAP Pharmaceutical Products representatives allegedly provided physicians with free samples of Lupron. They then allegedly helped several of these physicians obtain several hundred dollars' worth of government funds as a reimbursement for each alleged dose.

A third charge: according to a 2001 *New York Times* article by Melody Petersen, TAP Pharmaceutical Products representatives allegedly offered physicians "kickbacks," including "trips to resorts, medical equipment and money offered to the doctors as 'educational grants'" as incentives for prescribing Lupron.

Petersen details how TAP Pharmaceutical Products paid a settlement of $875 million, which was, at the time, the largest settlement for health-care fraud in the United States. According to their president, Petersen writes, TAP Pharmaceuticals chose to settle so as to not risk the possibility that the government would stop all reimbursements for Lupron. "We could not afford to have this drug denied to our patients," Petersen's article quotes him as saying. He also stressed that the case did not involve any questions of safety or efficacy.

84

AFTER MY BOWEL PUNCTURE, MY BODY HADN'T HAD LIQUID, much less solid, food in days. I started with water, a half paper cup at a time, then juice. I worried that my bowel puncture hadn't actually healed, that I'd begin leaking like a bad bicycle tire.

My first actual meal with something that resembled food was scheduled for the morning of Memorial Day. I walked the halls with my mother, one hand on my IV and another trying desperately to hold the back of my gown closed, even though my mother walked behind me to make sure nothing was exposed. It was important to walk, the nurses said. It was important to try and let my body find and gather strength. That day, the halls were emptier, the sounds softer, with smaller clusters of nurses around the soda fountain that dispensed Diet Coke, ginger ale, and ice water.

"Looks like the skeleton crew today," my mother said when we ambled our way out of earshot. "Good thing this isn't your first day." But it felt like my first day, like I'd been reborn into a world full of possibilities. The most important of these possibilities: a bowl of Cream of Wheat, which was to arrive on the wood laminate tray swung over the side of my hospital bed along with a cup of black coffee and, if I was lucky, a packet of sugar to sprinkle in both.

When a new nurse showed up with a bowl of Cream of Wheat, I thanked her four times in a row. I performed that hopeful hospital ritual of lifting the pink plastic hat whose job was to keep the contents of a pink plastic bowl hot. And then I shifted my focus to the contents of that pink plastic bowl, which looked strange for Cream of Wheat. At the same time too liquidy and too lumpy, somehow. I thought perhaps I was seeing things. I thought perhaps that it had made me hallucinate, this hunger, that it had nestled itself in so much of my being that I could no longer correctly determine the kind of food sitting in that plastic bowl in front of me. I dipped my spoon in, experimentally. I noticed and then told myself not to notice black flecks, like pepper.

"What," my mother said in the way that indicated she knew something was wrong from the way my face was arranged. I tried to relax the eyebrows that had, I'd realized, crept closer to each other.

"Well," I said. I stirred the Cream of Wheat and realized with an increasing conviction that it most definitely was not Cream of Wheat.

"What," my mother said, more definitively this time.

"This just looks a little like—funny." I couldn't say what I meant when I said *funny*, which was *gravy*. I meant *this just looks a little like gravy*.

"Well, it is hospital food." My mother craned her neck to look at the bowl and before she could look too closely, I took a bite. And it was gravy. It was indeed peppered white gravy, slopped into the bowl that was supposed to hold my first meal in five days.

"It's fine, it just—" I stopped myself. I couldn't lie to my mother, not with her neck craned toward the bowl, not with her nostrils, which I knew were sensitive enough to tell the difference between Cream of Wheat and gravy. "It kind of might be gravy?"

"Gravy?" Her voice leapt out, unexpected and strange as the taste I once again tasted when I put a second spoonful in my mouth. "Can't you tell?"

I could tell. I could absolutely tell. "No," I said in an unsure voice, a little high and weak at the edges.

"Emily Suzanne Bolden," she said, "do not eat that if that is gravy. You don't want to spend any more time here than you have to, and you'll have to if you eat gravy."

I dipped the spoon into the bowl again. I wanted to know how long I could keep this up, how long I could lie to my mother when she clearly knew I was lying. And here is the thing about hunger: it swallows everything. It contains all and it is impossible for it to be contained. It replaces every impulse, every want with the word *need*.

I put the spoon in my mouth. I imagined it touching every single taste bud. I imagined every single taste bud speaking back its thanks. I swallowed. "I think it's gravy," I said. "I think it's definitely gravy."

"What in the hell." Then my mother was out of her chair and the spoon was out of my hand and she was tasting what made my taste buds so grateful. "Who in the hell would bring you a bowl of *gravy*? This is a *cardiac floor*."

My mother took the bowl into the hallway. I knew she was talking to the head nurse, holding the bowl out under her nose and asking her to smell it. From my hospital bed, I could hear her hushed voice. I could hear anger spilling over the edges of that hush. At the same time, sickness rose in my stomach. I pushed the button on my Dilaudid pump, then watched the long hand of the clock begin its sweep through twenty minutes, like the nurses had taught me, until I could push the button again. When my mother returned, there was no bowl in her hand.

"They're bringing you Cream of Wheat," she said, "and that idiot nurse is never stepping foot in here again."

85

BECAUSE THE GYNECOLOGICAL SURGEON PUNCTURED MY bowel with his initial incision, he was not able to complete the exploratory surgery for which I had signed my consent. I therefore exited the hospital with more problems than before, since I had all the same old problems and the new problems of a punctured bowel and more adhesions. This meant that I could not have another exploratory laparoscopic procedure to clear my reproductive system and relieve my pain while preserving my fertility. It was too dangerous. The next surgical procedure would have to be a total hysterectomy.

On my fifth day in the hospital, the general surgeon who'd repaired my small bowel came to check on his work. He removed the bandages and examined my staples and incisions. I looked up at the ceiling. I did not want to examine my incisions. I did not even want to see his face as he examined my incisions.

My general surgeon declared that my whole-body was no longer at risk for sepsis. He called the team of nurses in to give them his instructions. Because the hospital was understaffed, it took a while for the nurses to come. In the meantime, he talked to my parents about bourbon. They told him that they liked Blanton's, but he suggested that they try Willett.

•

According to a 2009 article published in the *Journal of Gynecological Endoscopy and Surgery*, "bowel injury is the third cause of death from a laparoscopic procedure." The authors of the article performed a survey of approximately 37,000 gynecological laparoscopies performed in the United States. There was a 0.16 percent incidence of bowel injury, according to this survey.

The authors of this article refer to injuries occurring during laparoscopic procedures, including bowel injury, as "complications," which Wikipedia defines as "an unfavorable evolution of a disease, a health condition or treatment."

The term *unfavorable evolution* implies that something just happens, just like that. It implies that the thing that just happens, just like that, is out of anyone's control. It implies that everything that happened inside of my whole-body and all the ways that my whole-body was at risk were no one's fault. They were just a hazard of the game.

While the general surgeon waited for the nurses, he stood by the window and practiced his golf stroke. He held his arms and his hands the way that he would hold his arms and his hands if he were holding a golf club. He moved his legs away from each other until they stood in a wide stance. Then he turned his attention to his arms, which angled toward each other in a thin little isosceles of a triangle. He cocked his wrists and made a long, tall swing.

In other words, he executed a flop shot: a trick shot, one that golfers use in their most desperate circumstances. It's a variation of a chip shot that, if performed correctly, shoots the ball high over an obstacle and quickly brings it down. On the *Golf Digest* website, Dustin Johnson writes that the flop shot is "one of the game's ultimate risk-reward plays." If it fails, it fails miserably. But if it succeeds, it can quickly get a golfer out of trouble.

He executed it perfectly.

86

ON THE CURRENT LUPRON DEPOT FOR ENDOMETRIOSIS website, one reads, "In clinical trials, the most common side effects of LUPRON DEPOT, occurring in >10% of patients, include hot flashes/sweats, headache/migraine, decreased libido, depression/emotional lability, dizziness, nausea/vomiting, pain, vaginitis, and weight gain."

In the "What can you expect after discontinuing LUPRON DEPOT" section, patients are assured that "after completion of a full course of treatment with LUPRON DEPOT therapy, the hormonal effects you may have experienced should subside.[1]"

If one follows the superscript 1 to the bottom of the page, one will see that it refers not to a study or a peer-reviewed article, but to LUPRON DEPOT's very own packaging insert.

My parents' assessment of Willett, which they tried shortly after I got home: decent, but with a weird aftertaste, and not one they'd like to try again.

When I think about my time on the cardiac floor, I think about circles. The spheres of ice balanced against one another in the spoon's rounded bowl. The tiny ball trapped in a tube and the cycles of breath I used to blow into a mouthpiece in order to make it rise, in order to keep blood clots from clustering in my lungs. The route I walked down the hall and back, a parent on one side, a metal rack of machinery on the other, looped around the nurse's station. The hand I watched as it ticked its path around the clock and back again. Counting and hitting the red circle centered in the morphine pump's trigger. Waiting and counting again, until every trip around the clock flattened into the same spiral of time I moved in and moved in until I realized there was no such thing as starting or stopping, that circling was the whole of the story. Again. Again.

87

In a 2018 paper published in the *Journal of Pediatric & Adolescent Gynecology*, a group of Boston physicians detailed the results of their study to see if the use of GnRH agonists in adolescents with endometriosis caused long-term side effects. In the introduction, the authors describe how "the lay media" portrays such medications as dangerous. "Major media outlets publish stories of women with long-term, debilitating health problems that they attribute to use of leuprolide," they write. They mention the discussion forums and petitions that proliferate online. Nearly all the patients in their study experienced side effects during treatment, and 80 percent said these effects lasted over six months after their treatment concluded. Forty-five percent wrote that they'd experienced side effects they deemed "irreversible," including trouble sleeping, hot flashes, and problems with memory. Still, the authors of the study stress, the participants felt the medication was effective and would recommend it to other patients.

When I first read all the precautions and warnings about potential side effects for Lupron in 1998, the only words I understood were *some of which may not be reversible.* The other words seemed cryptic and coded: *asthenia, myalgia, peripheral neuropathy.* And because I didn't even know if there were online resources, I didn't sit at the computer and listen to the dial-up modem sing its song until Healthline or

WebMD or the Mayo Clinic's website loaded. I didn't type in each cryptic word so that I could be fully informed about what Lupron could do to me. I just folded the packet back up and put it in the trash can. I trusted the doctor. I trusted the drug.

By the time I was thirty-two, I didn't need a website to know what those words meant.

They meant that, every day, my body felt more like a strange thing, a coded and cryptic and strange thing that wasn't anything like me.

88

According to doctors like Freud and Charcot, when it comes to the story of their own bodies, women are unreliable narrators.

According to me, if this is true, it's largely because of doctors like Freud and Charcot.

THE TIGERS COME AT NIGHT

89

WHEN I WAS TWENTY-EIGHT, I SPENT THREE MONTHS listening to nothing but Feist's *The Reminder*, which I kept calling *The Remainder*. I made up for it by referring to Feist as Leslie Feist.

"Who the hell is Leslie Feist?" my friend Deena asked.

"You know, she did that 'one, two, three, four' song," I said.

"Oh, *Feist*. Just say *Feist*. Don't be a dick."

But sometimes I felt like I *wanted* to be a dick, like the times I felt too acutely aware of my floor as someone's ceiling and my ceiling as someone else's floor. I danced and sang anyway. Perhaps I wanted to be heard. For my neighbors to assume I was a woman happily dancing, gladly singing, with so many hopes she had to count them to keep them in order. In truth, time did a dance that turned the walls of my abdomen inside out.

My body housed a clock that I could hear, every moment, ticking. It had so many names: endometriosis, adenomyosis, polycystic ovary syndrome, pelvic adhesive disease. It was the year a doctor first discovered that a tumor had turned my uterine tissue into its home. It wasn't malignant, just a fibroid, but it was difficult to feel relieved. It was difficult to admit that, too. I just couldn't count my blessings.

A few weeks after the doctor found my fibroid, I printed out a photograph of (Leslie) Feist with her straight-perfect hair, holding up two fingers with two felt finger puppets: one a fox, one a raccoon. I gave the photograph to my stylist.

"Okay?" she said.

"Ignore the finger puppets," I said.

"The puppets aren't the problem. Your hair will not do this."

"I just like the shape of it," I said.

"It's a great haircut, but her hair is thin and straight and hangs flat, and your hair is thick and definitely not straight." She lifted the weight of it then let it half-fall, half-float in rebellion. "See?"

"I just like the *idea* of it," I said.

She sighed. She lifted her scissors. "I hope you have a heavy-duty straightener." She shook her head, but she made the first cut, as if in recognition that this was more about meaning than anything else.

During my second (Leslie) Feist–only month, a gynecologist referred me to a fertility specialist three hours away from the small college town where I was living. "This is beyond me," the gynecologist said. "It's beyond anyone I know around here," he said. "You need to see a specialist, and this doctor is known for working miracles." And so I drove three hours, listening to "I Feel It All" three times in a row, expecting a miracle.

I did not receive a miracle.

When I asked the fertility specialist if I could have children, he said he wouldn't say it was impossible, simply because, he told me, he never said anything was impossible. He said he was comfortable saying it was improbable. He said he was even comfortable with highly improbable. He said he was even comfortable with saying it would be impossible without intervention, without hormone shots and harvested eggs.

I asked him again. "I want to know," I said. "I need to know."

He laughed. He said, "I don't know, what's your husband's sperm count?" I told him I didn't have a husband. He laughed again. He said, "I know." By this he meant, *You're not even married, why are you asking me this?*

He said, again, that he wouldn't say it was impossible. He would say it was not likely. He would say that if I wanted to try, I'd better try sooner than later.

He said, "Even if you can conceive, it's likely that it would be difficult for you to carry a baby."

He said, "These answers might've been different when you were twenty."

He said, "Don't wait until you're thirty-eight and on your fifth PhD to realize you forgot to have a baby." By this he meant, *You have no right to ask*. By this he meant, *Lie down in this bed. You made it.*

90

In my late twenties, I worked as an instructor in my first faculty position. I was lucky because it was a full-time job, which meant I had benefits and a sense of security. I was unlucky because those benefits and that sense of security were guaranteed only for an absolute maximum of five years. It seemed strange, looking for a permanent relationship when the rest of my life was emphatically temporary.

Still, I could not, at any time—while preparing lectures on *The Iliad* for my World Literature I class or buying cinnamon crunch bagels at Panera or informing my cat that her efforts to pull loops of yarn out of my locker-hooked rug were not appreciated—forget that I was supposed to be trying to meet and love and marry someone so that I—that we—could have a baby.

I dated a man named Kennedy who taught in the same department as I did. We spent the last of summer arguing about *The Iliad* in a college bar in a college town abandoned by undergraduates. I bought the Marlboro Lights. He bought the gin and tonics.

They came in plastic cups with chipped ice and too much gin and made everything feel somewhere between absolute perfection and humiliation. I kept touching the lime then licking the bitter off of my fingers then touching the lime again. We smoked and we sat until the night became a string of Christmas lights pulsing at a rhythm that almost matched the rhythm of the music. It was almost beautiful. It was almost. And perhaps because of the almost-beauty, or perhaps because the beauty was always just almost, I didn't tell him about the morning that summer when I woke up and blinked and said "Oh" out loud to my feet, because they could not move.

One night I stayed with Kennedy in the bar until the music got louder and the night lost all its edges, lost all its perfect circles of light. Then we were laughing and walking and suddenly I felt very sure about the fact that there were stars above us. I laughed and the stars were there and we were walking and walking. Each glimpse of sky tasted like the space under my fingernails, which tasted like the lime.

He was wearing a gold chain and I hated it as we walked past the football stadium, past the huddled semicircles of apartments, past parking lots that bossed cars around with their white lines and squares. We'd been walking a very long time, so I said to him, "We've been walking a very long time?" I made it a question so he answered, "Almost there. Almost." He said it five more times—*Almost, almost. Almost. Almost almost*—and there were streets and sandwich shops and cars with the oldies station leaking out of closed windows.

When we stopped walking, we were in Kennedy's apartment. I sat on his couch and took off my shoes. I saw, with surprise, that both of my heels were bleeding. I hadn't felt pain. I hadn't felt anything. He was telling a story because he always told stories. And this story started the way that all his stories started, with an approximation of the characters' weights and heights, sometimes down to the half pound.

I made an *um-hm* noise. This was not a conversation. There was no need to respond further. I looked at my feet. I almost expected them to look back. I almost expected them to help me decide if I hated him and his almosts or not. I almost expected the big toe to move without my moving it. To nod to me, as if to say, *Oh no, honey. No.*

I kept looking at my feet and felt the way I felt sometimes when

I looked at them, as though they were strange and alien things, like not-quite-hands. Every time I thought that, I wondered if it was a strange thing to think. Because I'd actually thought it in front of someone, finally, I thought this could be my first and last chance. It was now or never. And so I asked, "Do you ever think of how feet are a very strange thing?"

He paused and made a noise in his throat, as though he was startled at my insouciance, which was the kind of word he would actually use. He said "anyway" a little too loudly and urgently, the way people do when a child interrupts them. When it's someone else's child, who they can't discipline.

91

As my body became larger and older, it became stranger and more complicated. It tripped and tumbled and stumbled and stuttered and stuck. It fell on sidewalks and in crosswalks and driveways, at public parks and Target superstores and, once, in the beer tent at a craft fair with my friend Deena, who was kind enough to pretend I was drunk and to half-shout, "That is *it*, my friend, I am cutting you off."

My body's arms flapped numbly. Its feet fired and needled. Its vision blurred and unblurred. Its skin felt and unfelt. By the time my body became twenty-five, I sometimes in my head told it to move and it told me no. It tripped. It tingled and pinned; it sent electric-feeling beats through its arms and hands and legs and feet, as though something inside of my nerves were dancing, singing. The wrong words. The wrong tune.

Kennedy kept telling his story. A woman in it wore a gray silk gown even though it was raining and she was famous, I guessed, because he used her first and last name and paused every time that he said it. I didn't recognize either the first or last name, so he made the noise in his throat and spoke too loudly and urgently again.

My feet felt strangely numb, like they weren't my feet, like they were as fat and blobbed as the feet I found under all my dolls' socks, with nothing but a few stitches to show where each toe ended and another began. I wondered, *What shade of gray silk? Clouds-building-a-summer-storm gray? Motor-oil-on-the-driveway gray?* It was like my feet weren't feet after all. Like they were, instead, age-spotted banana peels. Long and wet leaves, nibbled in places down to the netting of veins. An unhung hammock, slack and useless.

I tilted my head to the degree of casual curiosity. It looked enough like I was listening for him to keep talking, which made me feel safe enough to tap my feet against the carpet. And though I knew I was the one tapping the feet and that the tapped feet belonged to me, I didn't feel anything but a blank space where there should have been words, like *carpet, fabric,* and *floor.* It felt strange, so I kept tapping.

I kept tapping and feeling strange and curious. I didn't know, at that moment, that I should've been afraid about what was happening to my feet because I was too busy being afraid that I would never meet someone to love and marry and have children with before I was too old, before it was too late. I spent a lot of time thinking about that. I'd think of the word *old* and consider things: *No husband no child no permanent job no house no prospects either.*

Sometimes I thought, *My body is the trap from which I will not escape because the only way out is by death.* Sometimes I thought, *Well, that was dramatic. Jesus.* Sometimes I walked out of the Alehouse to smoke cigarettes in a circle of friends and realized with each step that I couldn't feel my legs, and it wasn't because they were asleep. Sometimes I clumsily paced the hallway of my apartment, up and down and up again, while talking to my parents on the phone, fighting to keep my voice level and calm and empty of evidence that my legs had simply stopped feeling. Sometimes I watched the clock when it ticked over to three in the morning, exactly, and I looked into those two red zeros while I wondered when the next episode would come and what I would do when and if it did, when and if I stopped walking completely, where I would go and who would take care of me. I didn't have plans. I had questions. There are no such things as answers.

•

Eventually, Kennedy's story ended. I made the *um-hm* noise again. I said, "Oh, wow." I said it as I was reaching for my shoes so I could go home and sit on my couch and shake my head at the walls and the cat for a while.

"Gosh, it's late," I said. He agreed. It was late, so we kissed for a few minutes, until I felt both satisfied and desperate. Then I was walking to the guest parking spots necklaced around the apartment's swimming pool, which looked as beautiful and eerie as every swimming pool does at night. And because I was thinking so much about how I had failed, yet again, to find someone to be in love with, I didn't pause to ask myself, *How many steps do I have left this time?* I didn't worry that my apartment didn't have a good guest bed because I didn't worry that my mother would have to come and live with me and do the things that living in one's own apartment requires—the swiffering and mopping, the grocery shopping, the folding and ironing and hanging up all the shirts and pants I slid off in dizzy exhaustion as soon as I got home from the job I worried I wouldn't be able to keep. I didn't feel the weight of this, the guilt of this, so heavy in the cradle of my rib cage, rocking. I just felt the cool of the night and its envelopes of stillness. I slipped into and out of them, toward and away from the sounds of strangers laughing and sputtering and trying to sing along to their stereos.

On the drive home, there were houses with lit windows and I looked inside of them. People were learning to live with one another. They were learning to talk and dance and cook. They moved into and out of the windows, which framed them as silhouettes, laughing with their heads tossed back, leaning in to speak softly to their telephones. And when I think of that night, I think of the woman I was in that half-price dress, and with the long hair that smelled like smoke and stiff hair spray, who moved everywhere,

everywhere, on those legs. I think of the football stadium and its open bowl of lights. I think of myself small beside it, my feet even smaller. I tell myself to keep walking. I tell myself to walk, as long and as far as I can.

92

I'M TWENTY-NINE, STILL BLURRY FROM SLEEP. I'M WATCHING a morning news show not by choice but because it's on the last channel I'd watched and I'm too tired to change it. I'm drinking coffee to wake myself enough to drive to the college where I teach freshman about the rhetorical triangle, when the girl I was in fifth grade appears on the screen.

Except the girl is nothing like me, in many ways. She's from Virginia, small for her age when I was always taller than my classmates, or, at least, the boys. She's got blond hair instead of my dark hair. It's a mess, though, like my hair always was; I can tell it was once cropped short but has grown out to an awkward length between shoulder and ear. She stands on legs like two too-thin pylons, keeping her body in sway. Her hand curls into a *C* under her freckle-crested nose as she sneezes. And this is when she becomes me, becomes the girl I was: she sneezes and sneezes and cannot stop, her body trapped in the same loop of motion that trapped my body when I coughed and coughed and couldn't stop.

I blink, rubbing my eyes. I wonder if I'm imagining things, if I'm so tired from grading and prepping and trying to stand steady in my low-heeled shoes while lecturing that I'm just imagining it, this girl whose body has betrayed her in such a familiar way. Then she sneezes again.

At first, it just seemed like the tail end of a cold. A stubborn sneeze. Now, she sees specialists—sometimes three or four a day. I imagine the stethoscopes, X-rays, tubes sent through her nose to her lungs. I imagine doctors' shoulders shrugged beneath white coats while her shoulders rise and fall and rise, sneezing at a rate of up to sixteen sneezes per minute, more than 20,000 sneezes a day. The girl stares, as if the sneeze is simply breathing, or a habit, like winding the tip of her hair around her index finger. She is desperate for a cure. Still they come, the sneezes as steady and placid and sure as words in their proper place in a sentence, as if her sneeze had become the steady company my own cough became.

She stares at a spot somewhere on the floor, where the camera's cables must lie, warmed and coiled. When an off-camera reporter asks how she feels about her unstoppable sneeze, she answers, prompt and polite, that she feels frustrated. Four sneezes pass between the words. I imagine that, like I did, the girl rests when her body rests. That she lies in bed and holds her breath to trick her chest to stop. In deep sleep, a sneeze is impossible: sleep lulls a person's motor neurons until they silence even the impulse of reflexes. Still, I imagine, she wakes to sneeze, filling the night's slurred quiet with sound.

93

WHEN MY BODY STOPPED FEELING AND MOVING THE WAY I asked it to, I did not want to take it to a specialist. I was tired of doctors. I was tired of living inside of a body that never seemed to work. I was tired of being told that this fact had little to do with the facts of my body, that it instead had to do with whatever had happened in my past, whatever was happening in my head. I told myself that what my body experienced could be explained, easily, by what doctors had already told me: the result of stress and exhaustion, or else the fibroid bulging from the back of my uterus, or else the enlarged uterus itself, or else endometriosis tangled in the net of nerves that travel to my legs. I did not want to think about another possible explanation: the Lupron shots I'd taken for far too many years, the treatment I myself had signed off on, and literally, with my sloppy signature in ballpoint pen.

And then the inexplicable found me: my arm lost its feeling. Entirely. I told myself I was writing by hand too much, then that I was typing too much. But after weeks of rest it was still without feeling, and almost without realizing it, I had told my mother.

It was winter break and I was ready to leave my grade book behind. I'd moved from a three-year temporary faculty position in Kentucky to a tenure-track position in Georgia only to find things were mostly the same. The same grade books and lecture notes. The same sense that nothing was permanent. The same serious colleagues trying to drink themselves out of seriousness at the same loosely organized faculty tailgates. The same closet full of broken-down moving boxes. My parents had driven from Alabama to Georgia to drive me and my hissing cats to their home for two weeks. That way, they could take turns driving and fighting over the radio while I sat in the back with the cats. There was more room in the back seat, more space for me to move my leg, to keep it from pain and pins and needles and numbness. That's why my parents insisted on driving: my right leg, which hadn't behaved like a leg for four years, which somehow cramped and throbbed and felt like nothing all at once.

That morning, I'd stuffed a tote bag full of all the things I'd planned to but probably would not read over the break. I knew the bag was heavy, bulging with hardback books. I'd shoved them in there myself. But when I slung the bag over my forearm, I couldn't feel it. I couldn't feel anything. I tried to arrange my face into an approximation of stillness, into the kind of expression that says *there is nothing at all wrong here, at all.*

My mother took one look at me. She knew. "What's wrong now?"

"I don't know," I said. I walked past her and out to the car. I tried to walk in a very quick way that said *there is nothing wrong here, if there were, would I be this fast at walking?* But she followed me with the same quickness, and so I said, "I can't feel my arm, I guess."

"You can't feel your *arm?*"

I shrugged. I shoved the book bag in the back of the SUV then shut the door with what I hoped sounded like a calm finality. "I don't know. It's been going on for a couple of weeks."

She looked at me and I looked at her. Neither of us said a thing. I got in the car, where my cats circled angrily inside of their carriers, meowing.

"Hush," I said to them and, by extension, to me. I didn't know why I had told her. I had made it real, and I was scared.

94

Within days of her interview, the girl who can't stop sneezing becomes a spectacle. A Reddit user posts a version of her video edited so that she sneezes 117 times in a minute. On a CNN segment, an expert discusses her symptoms. There are things we need to consider, he tells the viewer. Her sneezing stops at night. Her sneeze is not productive, which indicates that there is no actual irritation. The cause, the expert explains, is far more likely to be a "tic"—"psychogenic intractable sneezing," a disease which, a quick Google search reveals, is most common in young girls. The expert's words are played over footage of the girl sneezing and shaking and shuddering on a loop, sometimes edited to an impossible speed.

A reporter leans forward at his desk, curls his hands around his coffee mug. He asks the expert if he means that the girl's condition is psychological.

The expert stammers, qualifies his answer: She may have no idea what's happening. She may truly feel like she needs to sneeze. But yes, the expert agrees. The cause is psychological, not physical. He speaks over footage of the girl, sneezing and sneezing. I count fifty-one times.

My mother and I didn't talk about my arm for over a week. On one of my last days at home, we went to the Olive Garden. My mother tried to choose between the pizza and the eggplant parmigiana, which my father calls Eggplant Farmer John. I tried to choose between the Chicken Farmer John and some kind of mushroom ravioli.

"We're having chicken tonight," my mother said.

"Done," I said. When the waitress came, I ordered the ravioli.

"Tell me what you mean by numb," my mother said as we waited for the salad and breadsticks.

"I don't know," I said. "It's like when you go to the dentist and get Novocain. It feels like that. Like this," I said, and showed her the secret test I gave myself every morning, poking my limbs first with just my finger and then my fingernail. "I can't feel that at all."

"What do you mean you can't feel it?"

"I can't feel it. At all."

The wrinkle appeared between my mother's eyebrows, which meant that she felt worried. "Well, tell you what." She picked up a fork from her side of the table. "Can you feel this?" She poked my forearm with her fork.

I watched it and then looked at her. "No, I can't." She poked my hand. I winced. "I can feel there. Stop."

"So you can feel your fingers."

"Yeah."

"So that's good, at least."

"Yeah."

"You couldn't feel the other at all?"

"It's like when I had that thing done," I say, pointing to my lower abdomen, to the triangle just above my pubic bone. Seven years earlier, a plastic surgeon had deadened my skin then cut out a scar that, for six years, had swollen and bled and gotten infected from the endometriosis trapped inside. "It's like when you get local anesthesia. I can the feel pressure but not the pain."

My mother made her worried face and we both played with the gummed strips of paper that once held napkins over our silverware.

"Well," she said, "it's time to get this checked out. It's time to finally find out what's wrong."

"Yeah," I said. I slid my Diet Coke toward me on the table and lowered my head to sip from the straw. I'd been drinking Diet Cokes at restaurants like that for months. I tried to remember how many. I tried to remember when I'd realized why I drank that way: so I wouldn't have to pick up the glass. So I didn't drop the glass. So no one would notice, and it wouldn't be real.

Through most of the morning news segment, the Virginia girl sits next to her mother on a couch, arm against arm. Their bodies echo each other: arms folded, legs crossed, as if they are both sinking into themselves, though the daughter's body shakes and shudders with sneezes. Her life has stopped: no more school, no more playgrounds, little sleep. The mother is frustrated. The mother is frightened. But the mother will not stop until her daughter's sneezes do. It's her duty, her role. Still, she looks so tired. Cut to the mother on the couch alone. A living room without the lamps turned on. Late afternoon. She talks about how she can't reassure her child that things will improve, that the sneeze with disappear. Her voice breaks. It is clear that she's at the edge of crying. It is clear that she will not let herself cry. The camera keeps its eye steady, servile and wide.

That night, my mother cooked dinner—chicken, as she'd promised at the Olive Garden, and roasted asparagus that tasted the way I can never make roasted asparagus taste. She stood by the stove, spearing spears of asparagus from their pan and chewing them while my black cat circled her legs to beg.

"Shoo, Gertrude," my mother said, and my cat jumped into my

lap, where she sat and purred and looked through the underside of the glass table at which my father and I ate what she wanted to eat. "I'm not going to miss that cat when you go home."

"You don't have to," I said, "she's staying here."

"No way," my father said, putting down his tea. "We're getting an English bulldog and naming it Winston Churchill."

"No way." My mother took the empty pans to the sink.

We were trying to remember when it started, the numbness, or if there was a when.

"Do you remember anything? Like lifting anything and hurting yourself?" My father cut the last of his chicken and Gertrude purred harder, like a question.

"That damn book bag." My mother turned on the faucet, then put her hand underneath it, waiting for the water to warm to hot. "Every time she flies in it's so heavy I can't carry it. I told her that'd mess up her back, but she never listens."

"I'm sitting right here, you guys. I can hear you." I felt Gertrude's claws in my lap, which meant she wanted to jump onto my father's lap. I held her back with both hands. "I don't remember anything."

My mother jerked her hand from the water, then put a pan in the sink. "But you've never had trouble with that arm."

I looked down at my plate and my father's almost-empty plate. My plate sat almost full. Every Thanksgiving, I was the last one at the table, chewing the turkey while my cousins cut into the German chocolate cake. I thought about this instead of what I should be saying to my mother, and then I was saying it, carefully, or it was saying itself, like it had been waiting, like the words themselves had been holding my tongue. "I've been dropping things for a while. I always think I have my keys, then they're on the floor."

My mother wasn't looking at me. I wasn't sure I was even talking. She looked at the sink. Steam clouded around it. My father made the face he makes when he's thinking. My cat's head appeared at the table's edge, making the face that she makes when she smells something she wants to steal or to kill.

"You need to make that cat stop begging," my mother said.

"Tell me about it." I nudged her face away. "I can't remember when it all started," I said, which was true. I spent a lot of time telling myself that nothing had started. I told myself that was the truth. "It's just a lot of little stuff that's happened over time, I guess. I guess it's kind of built up is all."

My mother turned off the water and walked to the table. She picked up the aluminum pan with its circle of rolls, the butter dish, my father's empty plate. She didn't look at them or anyone. She put the rolls on the countertop, the plate and the butter dish in the sink. I focused on forking the asparagus, perfectly, so that the four fork holes stood together in line. Then I heard the sound of crying. By the time I looked up, my mother had braced herself against the counter. Her elbows were locked. I dropped my fork.

"It just can't be anything bad," she said. "It just can't be MS. It can't be." My father stood up and then he was holding her, and then I was watching them hold each other. My mother cried into my father's Alabama Crimson Tide championship T-shirt. I knew from the sound that she was crying hard. My right arm, heavy and unfeeling, sat useless in my lap. I looked at it and at my cat, who looked at me, then nudged my hand. I didn't feel anything.

"I'm okay," I said. I was not crying. "I'm okay. I'll be okay. And maybe it'll be a good party trick? Stick a fork in me? I'm done?"

"That isn't funny," my mother said into my father's shirt. "That isn't funny." He patted her on the back and looked at the cabinets. I imagined that if he were looking at me, he'd be raising his eyebrows to tell me it was, actually, funny.

"I know," I said. "I'm trying."

95

In a 2006 segment on NPR's *Weekend Edition*, Linda Wertheimer and her guest, Elaine Fantham, talk about the way the ancient world viewed sneezing. The ancient Greeks, for instance, saw the sneeze as a prophecy. Once Xenophon, an Athenian general, roused men to horse, arrow, and sword not with words but with a soldier's incidental sneeze. An hour's worth of rhetoric from Xenophon could not convince his troops to rise, but when one of their own sneezed, they bowed and strapped their armor tight, inspired and assured of their safety.

Homer writes that Penelope didn't at first know her disguised and far-wandered husband, didn't recognize the color of his eyes, the familiar shift of his gait. She saw him as the stranger he'd become, not as the wish she wove all those nights into the death shroud she unraveled when morning arrived and he did not. She told Odysseus that her husband would soon return to challenge each suitor, her hands following the warp and weft of thread on the loom. Then their son, Telemachus, sneezed behind her. In the echo of the sound, she saw the stranger as her husband: the curve of the forehead she'd traced each morning in early light, the curved scar a boar's tusk left behind. Before the sound took its echo and left, she knew him. He was hers. She gave her body to his arms.

Later, in Europe's Middle Ages, the sneeze was seen as a danger. They believed that life was knotted to breath so tightly that such a great burst of breath could only bring harm, and so they chanted *God bless you*: an earnest Christian prayer.

96

BECAUSE MY PARENTS ASKED ME TO, I TOOK MY BODY TO many doctors who asked it to do many things. To push their hands away. To stand on one foot and then on the other. To feel the needles pressed into its skin. My body said no, and so the doctors put it into machines. They used magnets and radio waves to take a picture of the inside of my body. Because they'd seen the outside of my body move in the wrong ways, they expected to find the wrong things inside of my body. Specifically, they expected to find lesions on my brain and spine. In other words, they expected the images to confirm that I had relapsing-remitting multiple sclerosis, as my patient history and neurological exams had.

The images did not confirm that I had relapsing-remitting multiple sclerosis, and so all my many doctors pushed up their shoulders and sent my body to other doctors, like children saying *Idon'tknowIdon'tknow*.

In the morning news segment interview, the Virginia girl describes how she has trained herself to eat in only tiny doses—I imagine two peas at a time, the tip of a carrot—so she won't choke when her body does what it must. I imagine her family has given up on *God bless you*. They sit around the dinner table, looking at their plates instead of one another.

It takes a year for doctors to give the girl a name and a reason for what is happening to her body: a streptococcal infection gone wrong, or else misidentified. PANDAS, or pediatric autoimmune neuropsychiatric disorder associated with streptococcal infection: an autoimmune condition in which the body's defenses become too confused and distracted to fight bacteria, turning instead to the brain itself, antibodies latching onto neurons. I feel a jealous anger when I hear she's been given a reason with a name. I feel guilty when a doctor explains that reason further, explains that a child with this condition can sneeze as many as 12,000 times per day. The child can develop Tourette's syndrome, attention deficit disorder. The child can argue without knowing she's arguing, can shout obscenities without even choosing to. The child can move without moving herself, her arm or leg or chest caught up in a tic, twitching or hitting her own body in violent pantomime.

The child cannot be cured.

In interviews, the mother is glad her child's illness has a name, has a treatment. The mother says her child is better. The mother knows it may not last. I hear her voice tearing at the edges, exhaustion-thin. Her eyes are ringed with sleepless red. Still, the girl's body performs, moves through its motions and says what neither of them nor the doctors will say: *This flesh is not my flesh, this self not under my control.*

97

I FOUND MYSELF ALONE. THE BEGINNING OF OCTOBER. I opened the door to the linen closet and looked at the silver box in which my Halloween decorations—a plastic jack-o'-lantern with an electric candle, an arched black cat nearly identical to my own arched black cat—lived. I closed the door. Then I was on the couch and shaking very hard. I couldn't tell if I was very cold. I pulled a quilt over my body until I sank almost entirely under its surface. I shook in a way that made my cats puffer-fish up and glide away. I listened to my teeth. I stared at the television, which stared blankly back. I shook and shook.

When I became able to move my head, it was only in tiny clock-ticks to the right. I looked at the window and realized I'd forgotten to close the blinds, which felt embarrassing. I turned on the television so my neighbors would see that I had a reason for sitting on the couch beyond shaking. I didn't watch it. Instead, I counted to myself, slowly, and sometimes with a *Mississippi* between each number, until the pain broke long enough for me to walk to my bedroom. It felt more like sliding. I kept one hand on the wall.

I took my body to eight years' worth of doctors before a neurologist told me what might've gone wrong inside of it. Though that thing isn't wrong, exactly. It isn't incorrect. It isn't singing the lyrics of "No Woman, No Cry" to the tune of "Don't Rock My Boat." It isn't the

answer *Madonna* to the question *Who is on the quarter?* It is instead
something that is missing. Or, rather, something that never arrived,
like a postcard mailed to Canada with only one American Forever
stamp.

Here is what the neurologist told me: when human beings are
embryos, our spinal cords aren't cords. What will become the spinal
cord is a sheet of tissue, postcard flat. When our bodies change from
embryos into fetuses, the postcard-flat sheet of tissue rolls itself into a
tube. A proper metaphor for this may be: the construction paper you
as a child rolled up to use as a periscope. A telescope. The Thanksgiving issue of *Southern Living* magazine you rolled up and put to your
eye so you could look through all that orange and say, *Argh argh.* This
tube looks like a canal. It channels cerebrospinal fluid through the
center of the spinal cord, which was such a good simile that doctors
decided to call it the central canal. The central canal of most human
bodies closes completely as the human becomes larger and older.

The central canal of my human body did not close completely,
the neurologist told me, even when I became larger and older. And
so there are all these holes inside of it, all these very small holes, like
the empty spaces in the crocheted yarn that becomes a blanket, a
seemingly solid thing.

For a very long time, the neurologist explained, doctors thought
that holes in a person's spinal cord were just small-in-the-sense-of-
harmless incidental things. Even with the holes, they thought, the
body was still a whole fabric, a fully functioning thing. But the more
that doctors matched up the pictures of a person's body and the things
that went wrong when that body moved—the falling, the dizzying,
the clumsying—the less incidental the holes seemed. The less small.
The less asymptomatic. And so, he said, an unclosed central canal was
a disorder. Even if it didn't have a name, it was a real thing.

I did and did not believe him.

I do and do not think he was right.

I walked out of his office and to my car, my head down so I could watch the ground, so I could ready myself for shifting, for shaking, for falling. I told myself not to be afraid of driving simply because I had no choice but to drive—there was no one to drive me. I used my cell phone as an excuse for looking down. I wondered, for a moment and not for the last time, if maybe the neurologist too had felt desperate, if maybe he also just wanted some way for the things that happen in my body to be explained. I texted my friend Deena, *So my body is messed up because there are holes in my spinal cord?*

She texted back, *Like a flute?*

And I texted back, *Yes actually like a flute.* And then Deena texted, *SPINEFLUTE.* And I knew we were moving through different places in different kinds of light and both looking at our phones and laughing, guilty-laughing, at the language we had made.

By the time the neurologist found the holes in my spine, the calendar had made its way to almost-Halloween. Someone had taped a skeleton on the door of the bathroom. He helloed his finger bones and smiled his jawbone in the waiting room's direction. The skeleton could've belonged to a person about my height, if the skeleton were not two-dimensional and made of card stock. The skeleton was silver-prism-shiny and also almost falling off, as the tape that connected his skull to the door had vanished, much like his muscles, nerves, and skin. Anywhere else, it would've seemed funny, an appropriate companion for pumpkins and black cats with fear mohawks spiking their spines. But in the neurologist's office, it seemed like a very bad joke. A reminder that we were all haunted by something inside of our bodies and outside of our control.

98

A Saturday. September. Another loosely organized faculty football tailgate. We grilled sausages and sat in foldable fishing chairs and tried to pretend we weren't constantly aware that our own students sat a few foldable fishing chairs away. I sat between a man named Brig, whose research involved statistics about prisons, and my former-enemy-now-friend Cassandra. Cassandra and I hated each other when we first met—or, at least, I assumed she also hated me—for reasons I no longer remember and therefore assume boiled down, on my part, to jealousy.

Cassandra was brilliant, a philosopher who studied how the physical elements of human behavior evolve in an increasingly digital world. She was beautiful, too, and always seemed so confident in her sleek black hair and sleek tight jeans. I don't remember how we stopped being enemies and start being friends, either, except that we somehow agreed to watch *The Hunger Games* together in a movie theater that served beer and ridiculous burgers, holding hands and crying as Rue died.

At the tailgate, we did what we did at every tailgate. We downed beers perfunctorily and laughed at the clusters of girls marching in matching outfits to the bathroom and back, linking arms and singing, losing the lyrics as they weaved and walked. We drank until we got drunk enough to smoke and pretend this was a surprise, even though we'd all brought cigarettes. Afterward, we went to Brig's house. There, we clustered together in his garage to drink and smoke, the door open three inches.

Around my fourth beer it occurred to me that I might make out with Brig. Then we were the last people at the house. His mouth covered my mouth and I realized I was right. We had had a lot of fun, which is the word I guessed one used to describe a time that, in the company of a large group of people, one consumed large amounts of alcohol.

When I started dating, I did this terrible kind of math every time I got serious about someone, which was basically every time I went on a date with someone. Every day brought me closer to the limits of my own (1) fertility and (2) ability to function within a body that wouldn't stop stopping me, wouldn't stop shaking, wouldn't stop making pain. Every date drew out an equation that could lead to a solution: me as a wife, my date as a husband, and a variable determined either by a factor of XX or XY as our child. Dating was never about the possibility of sex for me, and sex was only about the possibility of having a child before I had to have a hysterectomy. I thought that was the most beautiful solution. I had been taught that way.

"You *made out*?" Cassandra said when I told her what happened between Brig and me. "What are you, in eighth grade?"

"What else am I supposed to call it?"

"I don't know," Cassandra said, "maybe, like, foreplay? You're a grown woman, you can talk about it." But the truth is that I didn't like talking about it. And I didn't like making out in the first place, for a general set of reasons: other people's mouths always tasted strange; I hated the way stubbled skin felt against mine; I was always aware of the stubble on my own legs and armpits. Plus, I wasn't sure if what Brig and I did qualified as foreplay, as there was no play to follow.

Even so, when I was with Brig, my body was occupied. Distracted. My body had a job to do. And it was easier to think about my body in this make-out-specific situation than to think about my body in general. My body in general and I had reached an impossible impasse. Constant periods. Constant shock waves of abdominal pain. Sometimes, when I walked, my legs worked just fine, thank you. Sometimes I'd be walking through a parking lot or on a sidewalk, moving just fine, thank you. And then I wouldn't be walking. My body and I, downed. My mother worried. Every other phone call ended with the same plea: "Emily, you need to go through your closet. You need to give those high heels away. You're going to really hurt yourself one day."

With Brig, my focus narrowed to one moment. To one now. To lying with him on a mattress on a floor covered in almost-colorless, sweat-smelling sheets, Axe body spray cans lined up in military precision in his bathroom, fifteen steps away.

Though the variables and constants changed, a standard formula for the Bolden Offspring Equation remained:

I am __ years old. If I date Man __ for __ years before we get married, and if Man __ and I are married for __ years before we produce biological offspring, I will be able to produce a biological offspring before I am age __.

Examples of solutions for the Bolden Offspring Equation include:

I am 25 years old. If I date Man A for 2 years before we get married, and if Man A and I are married for 2 years before we produce biological offspring, I will be able to produce a biological offspring before I am age 30.

I am 28 years old. If I date Man B for 1.5 years before we get married, and if Man B and I are married for 1.5 years before we produce biological offspring, I will be able to produce a biological offspring before I am age 32.

I am 30 years old. If I date Man C for 1 year before we get married, and if Man C and I are married for 1 year before we produce biological offspring, I will be able to produce a biological offspring before I am age 33.

All algebraic iterations of the equation had the same solution: panic. What would happen if my math failed, if I simply could not wait?

Here is a list of similes I used to describe dating against a deadline to my mother, in order of increasing desperation.

- It's like shopping for shoes that are both comfortable and attractive enough for a wedding: some pairs don't fit, some blister your heels, but if you're patient and keep your faith in quality footwear, you'll find the pair that's meant for you.
- It's like playing musical chairs with Marvin Gaye on the turntable: it's fun and exciting, dizzyingly so, until everything in the room—the music and the chairs and the inhaled air and the exhaled air and the men and most of all you—are blurred beyond function and belief.
- It's like a box of chocolates: everything tastes like disappointment and you become a cliché.
- It's like a backward game of Russian roulette: you're trying for the one chamber without a round to kill you.

99

AROUND THE THIRD OR SO WEEK THAT BRIG AND I FOUND ourselves making out with each other, I put on that sheer Swiss dot blouse—a careful white camisole beneath—and the gold necklace with a birdcage that carried inside of it a small gold bird, and those bell-bottom jeans. They were too long and required a high heel so that they wouldn't drag the ground while I walked. I crouched in front of my closet, eye-to-eye with the shoes standing in left-right pairs on my shoe tree, then pulled out the tallest pair of shoes I had. Wooden soles with three-and-a-half-inch heels. I strapped my feet into them. I stood. My ankles shifted in opposite directions, as if they were clearing their throats the way people do when you're about to embarrass yourself.

I ignored them.

I walked with a measured confidence out of my duplex and to my Toyota Matrix, which I drove to Brig's house. It was after his night class, early autumn, and the trees were just starting to lose the loose fabric of their leaves and reveal themselves as bony, eerie limbs. When he came to the door, he kissed me. I returned the gesture.

"So where do you want to go?"

"I don't know," I said, "you pick."

"Panera," he grumbled, "what the hell." We walked from his front door down the pathway to his car, through the darkness hanging down in its strange early autumn ways. He walked ahead of me, focused on reading someone's text on his phone. I worried, I wondered—was it his ex? Sometimes she drove across state lines to put a week's worth of casseroles in his freezer. She owned an actual apron, I was sure of it, and actually used it and also kissed him not as gesture of politeness but as something raw and open, an entrance into another kind of light and life. Every detail I knew about her was a reminder of who I wished I could be: A good sexual partner. A good wife. A mother.

I stood there, hating her. And then I wasn't standing anymore.

Brig wasn't looking, thank God, when I fell. Instead, he stood by the driver's side door, which he had politely opened for me, which stood between him, thank God, and me. I pretended to casually sit on the driveway. I watched the top of his head rotate, scanning the driveway and yard.

"Where did you go?"

I swallowed. I wiped the tears from under my eyes in a careful way that, I prayed, kept my mascara in place. I breathed into a calm voice and said, "Oh, I decided I'd just sit down on the sidewalk for a minute."

"You did?" He walked to my side of the car, head tilted, and looked at me in the way I imagined he looked at a row of data that defied his expectations.

"No." I tried to sound casual. "I fell and this is incredibly embarrassing."

"Yeah, there's that crack there." He gestured to a point on the driveway that I knew, beyond a doubt, was nowhere near the spot where I'd fallen. "Gets people all the time."

"That must have been it." I tried to say it with the confidence of someone who knows, beyond a doubt, that she was tripped by that crack that got people all the time. He stood for a while and I sat for a while and we both looked back at that crack.

"Well," he said, "are you going to just sit there? Should I bring you a sandwich or something?"

"Ha ha," I said. I put both of my hands down and pushed myself up. Except I didn't stand. I moved myself maybe an inch and a half, at the maximum. Pain lightninged through me. "Well, shit," I said. Brig walked over, extending one hand and then another hand, and pulled me up until I was standing. Sort of. I was stand-leaning. I moved my left leg forward. I tried to put weight on it. And then pain. It felt like what I imagined people meant when they used the phrase *bone against bone*, something that felt synonymous with the word *grind*. "Jesus," I said.

"You need me to get you a wheelbarrow or something?" It was just the way we flirted with each other, I told myself, like we didn't like each other when we really did. Still, I couldn't help myself. I glared. He held his hands up and apart and waved them. "Okay, okay. No wheelbarrow. Just trying to help."

"I am fine," I said. "I do not need help."

I was not fine. I did need help. But I also, I told myself, needed to go on this date, needed to show him that I was strong. Resilient. The kind of girl who could just keep going and going, without help, even if I couldn't cook casseroles. I shifted my weight to my nongrinding foot and hopped forward. And so I made it into the car and out of the car and into Panera. Through a cup of baked potato soup. From Panera's door to his car to his door and then down his hallway. To his bedroom. To his bed. I did my best to kiss him back and make hopefully pleasurable sounds. When he tried, as always, to go further, I pushed him backward, as always. He got out of bed and put on his filthy blue bathrobe.

"That looks like the skin of a sick Muppet." I swung my feet over the side of the bed. "It's late," I said.

"It's late," he agreed. I thanked him for dinner. I felt like I always felt on dates, as if there was some unwritten rule that it was time for me to have sex with him and he blamed me with a righteous anger for not doing so. Perhaps I felt guilty. Perhaps that's why I didn't ask for his help. I hopped down his hallway with my shoes in my hand, the hem of my jeans under my feet, until he said, "What, are you practicing the pogo stick?" Perhaps that's why I didn't tell him to go to hell, that if he wanted someone to screw that much he should just go ahead and screw himself.

By the next morning, I could no longer pretend that I was fine. I drove myself to the doctor's office and there, three steps from my car, I reached my limit. I couldn't walk. I couldn't hop. I couldn't move forward at all. A man came out, saw me, and immediately went back inside to get a wheelchair.

"There's this little hump between the ankle and the heel bone called the talus bone," the doctor said, pointing to an illustration of the foot. "Your talus bone is broken. In half. Completely."

"Holy crap," I said. The doctor nodded.

"This is a very unusual kind of injury. Usually we see it in snowboarders or skiers, or people who've been in high-impact crashes," he said. He shook his head. "How did this happen?" And so I told him: the driveway and the crack I knew, even as I said it, hadn't tripped me at all, the car and the dinner and the hopping, pogo-stick-like. He furrowed his brow and shook his head, slowly, from side to side.

"Was it a good date, at least?"

"You know what? It wasn't." I listened to my own words and surprised myself, and so I laughed a little. "It definitely was not worth this."

100

IT TOOK TWO WEEKS FOR BRIG AND I TO STOP SEEING EACH other.

It took four months for my foot to heal.

I decided I needed to meet new people. To get out more. I decided that if there was a time for me to bloom fully into the life of the body, this was it. And so when Cassandra asked if I want to go to the new faculty mixer, I heard the surprise in her voice when I said yes.

"Woah," Cassandra said when she picked me up, "I didn't know this was a formal occasion." I wore a bright striped halter dress with a white short-sleeved sweater for modesty. She wore skinny jeans and a short-sleeved red sweater and looked more phenomenal and confident than I could ever be.

"Every occasion is a formal occasion if you want it to be," I said.

"You are the master of fashion," she said. We headed to the half of campus we never saw, the science buildings where the faculty made starting salaries higher than we'd ever reach. All I could think or talk about was the prospect of seeing Brig and, possibly, the woman I assumed he was making out with now.

"I could just pretend like I need to pee," I told Cassandra. "I could hide in the bathroom."

"Dude. Do *not* hide in the bathroom."

"It's safe in the bathroom."

"You are *not* going to hide in the bathroom. You are going to stand there with your head high and make him remember how lucky he was that he got to make out with you."

"Okay," I said, "I guess that's true," even though I really guessed the opposite. "I am not going to hide in the bathroom."

"Just say hi and then pretend there's someone more important you want to talk to."

"I can do that," I said, looking out the window at the college bars and fast-food drive-throughs. "I can totally do this."

As soon as we got out of the car, I knew: I totally could not do this. I picked up a glass of white wine before I Sharpied my name onto the name tag stickers fanned across the table. I finished half of the glass before I'd smoothed the sticker onto my dress. Within ten minutes, I began to feel my palms in that way that let me know I was buzzed and on my way to drunk.

101

THIS IS THE STORY I THINK I REMEMBER. THIS IS ALSO THE story that might be wrong.

I didn't see Brig. Then I did. He was standing at the free wine table beside me. Cassandra was in the bathroom or somewhere, I can't remember, and I became intensely aware of my cheeks and arm-pits and the fact that my body temperature had risen to an alarming degree. I became intensely aware of myself as a stack of loosely con-nected bones and flesh standing next to another stack of bones and flesh who had, unfortunately, seen me braless in Hanes Her Ways.

I think I remember that Brig said hello in a way that could have indicated interest or boredom. I gave him a sharp little nod and a *hi* and hoped it didn't sound as if I were actually literally melting, which is exactly what I (1) felt like I was doing and (2) most wished I could do. I asked how he was doing. He said, "Fine," and then asked how I was doing. I said, "Fine." I looked a little past him and made a gesture that I hoped implied I'd found a group of people I liked more than him, a stack of bones and flesh wearing one of eighteen varieties of Axe body spray.

"Have a good semester, Brig." I took two glasses of wine from the table. I couldn't remember how many glasses I'd already had. That did not give me pause. I didn't wait to see if he'd say *goodbye* or *you too* or *can we have more of a conversation and then several more glasses of wine at my house?* I *excused me*'d and *sorry*'d my way through the crowd until I'd made my way to the hallway outside the women's restroom. I chugged both glasses of wine.

The night blurred by.

The faculty members blurred by, too, in their dress-casual button-ups and dark-wash jeans and midlength dresses and glasses. My ankles wavered every time I walked and so all my focus and concentration went into walking. *Don't fall don't fall don't fall*, I said to myself in my head, focusing so intently that I stopped speaking entirely. I didn't realize I'd been silent until Cassandra under-her-breath asked if I was okay.

"Brig," I under-my-breath told her.

"That asshole," she out-loud said, then scanned the room for him. "He must be gone," she said, but I still couldn't start talking. I still couldn't stop sweating and blushing and standing there in alarm as my ankles wavered toward surrender, and all I could think was that this whole room full of new faculty members might see me fall, face flat, legs splayed, showing my Hanes Her Ways.

102

I DON'T REMEMBER WHY WE WENT TO CASSANDRA'S apartment before she took me home. I do remember, and with certainty, her and me and Priam, her Boston terrier, on the lawn behind her apartment. I stood as still as possible, smoking a Marlboro Light I'd hidden in the zipper pouch of my purse in the hope that it would make me sober. It absolutely did not make me sober. Instead, it made my head feel very heavy and light at the same time, like a weighted balloon, and I started to feel the acid creeping up my throat. I started to panic and told myself to stop. To stop being drunk. To stop smoking. To stop being so utterly messy all the goddamn time. Cassandra was kind enough to stand there, Priam's leash in her hand, as if I stood and acted the way I'd always stood and acted on that scrap of lawn, talking quietly and waiting for her dog to pee.

I don't remember when I knew I was going to be sick. "I don't feel so good," I'm sure I said, maybe after Priam had finally done what we'd come out here for him to do, maybe after I'd made it to the filter of my cigarette, maybe as we made our loud and careful way up the two flights of stairs to her apartment. I don't remember walking through the door of the apartment or the door to the bathroom. I just remember the lights and the cold of the tile as I kneeled in Cassandra's guest bathroom and, as quietly as possible and while crying, I threw up. Over and over again.

Cassandra knocked gently on the door, asking if I was okay, saying, "Oh God that does *not* sound good," asking if I needed anything, like some water maybe? I might have said no. I definitely said, "I'm sorry," over and over. *I'm sorry I'm so sorry I'm sorry.* Like it was a prayer or song or chant. When I'd taken a break from throwing up, I heard Cassandra knock again.

"Girl, you do not want to see this," I said.

"Girl, I'm not looking," she said, and then the door opened, just enough for her hand to come through. She held out a glass of water. "Drink this," she said. "It'll make you feel better."

And I did feel better, for a while, until I started throwing up again. I started rehearsing all my usual excuses. It was medication. It was my period or my acid reflux. It was the pain I carried around with me all the time in my abdomen. It was so hot and I was so nervous and that must have been it. I did not think: *Maybe it was the two glasses of wine you chugged, or the however many you drank before that, or the cigarette you smoked past the filter.*

I don't remember how long I was on Cassandra's bathroom floor. I do remember that I cleaned her toilet and tile and sink. Four times. I opened the bathroom door, cautiously. "I'm okay, I think," I said. "But I used up your Clorox wipes."

"Did you clean the bathroom?!"

"Four times. It should be clean."

"Dude," she said, poking her head into the bathroom door. "You're completely insane. You didn't have to do that. But thank you."

103

I STARTED HAVING THIS DREAM.

I'm standing, bassinet-side, my palm cupping the small skull of a baby. Its skin is soft, like the peach-fuzzed skin of the doll I once hugged before sleeping each night, pressing my cheek to the plastic of its cheek. In the dream, I press my cheek against the baby's cheek. It is morning, and I hold the baby to the sun, which slides in through valance, curtain, blind. Light settles kindly and clearly on the blue walls of the room. It's painted like a sky, ceiling circled with clouds circling the light fixture, a sun. I dream that the sun is a spotlight on the baby's shining, sleeping face. The dream is perfect. Then it is terrible. The baby's cheeks collapse and cave in, as if someone held a magnifying glass between it and July's brute beast of a sun. The baby melts and shrinks to the size and shape of an egg, flesh-colored, speckled red, the exact same shape and size as the tumor the doctors saw growing in my uterus, settled in its relentless restlessness.

I try and can't remember, can't decide if I trust my own memory: Did I really see Brig at the reception, or do I tell myself that I saw him, to justify how I behaved, how much I drank?

•

I decided to try out an excuse on Cassandra during the drive back to my duplex. I wanted to see if she believed me. I wanted to see if I could say it well enough to be believed.

"I'm so sorry about that," I said. "I'm just on my period and I've been on this new medicine and I just got so nervous, you know?"

"I know," she said. "I know. But all that wine probably didn't help either, lady," she said. "You hit it a little hard tonight." And I laughed a little because she was right, and because she had said it out loud. I felt a little better. I felt a little like I could be better because there in the driver's seat was a person who cared about me enough to crouch down and reach through the bathroom door with a glass of water, who cared enough about me to know when I was lying, to know what I was avoiding, and to say something I needed to hear.

104

In Greek mythology, Cassandra was a princess of Troy, the daughter of King Priam and Queen Hecuba, blessed by the gods with the gift of prophecy but, at the same time, cursed: she would always speak the truth, and the mortals who listened would never believe her. As always, myth offers different stories to explain why. In some, Cassandra promised Apollo her love in exchange for the gift of prophecy. When she didn't give him her love, the god cursed her with the fate that she would never be believed. In other stories, Cassandra didn't ask for her powers. She didn't barter an exchange. Instead, Apollo granted her the gift because he thought she'd love him; when she didn't love him for his gift, he gifted her with a curse. In still other stories, the gods weren't involved at all. Instead, snakes flicked their forked tongues in her ears so that they heard the future.

Whatever the particular details of the story, the meaning remained the same: Cassandra spoke the truth, and those around her may have heard, but they never believed. When the Greeks rolled their great horse to the walls of Troy, Cassandra told the Trojans that there were armed men waiting, sharpening their swords in the great dark belly of the wooden beast. The Trojans ignored her, and so the gift they saw as a sign of their own greatness instead brought their own downfall.

•

Cassandra and I met at Ruby Tuesday for lunch. She had a beer and I had a lavender pear martini. A lavender tea bag floated in the middle of my drink, coloring it red.

"Doesn't this look a little like a tampon?" I asked with scrunched-up lips.

Cassandra scrunched her lips in echo. "Ew. And definitely." I took the tea bag out and let it bleed over my bread plate.

"Anyway," I was saying, "it just—I don't know. I mean, even if I could somehow have a baby, what happens if my arms go numb and I can't hold it? Or what if I manage to pick it up, then drop it?"

Cassandra made a sound that sounded like *gosh* and for a minute her eyes seemed very wet. Then she said, "I mean," and turned her beer a half turn on its cardboard coaster, on which was printed a picture of the same beer she was drinking. "That is just so sad," she said, "and I totally get it. I get it. This sucks to think about, but I think you're thinking in a very mature way."

105

WHEN I WAS THIRTY-ONE, I STARTED TALKING TO A gynecologist about a hysterectomy.

Six months later, I met a man. He'd interviewed for a job at the university where I spent most of my time telling my poetry classes to show, not tell. He got the job, and in the months before his old job ended and his new job began, we talked on the phone. Sometimes for six hours a day.

"Sometimes I feel like I know him better than anyone I've ever known," I told Cassandra, but only after our second glass of wine.

"Maybe wait until you're actually living in the same city," Cassandra told me, but only after our third glass of wine.

It was true. Sometimes I felt like I knew him better than anyone I'd ever known. I also knew him very little, if at all. Half of myself tried to convince the other half that falling in love with him was a terrible idea, and half of myself tried to convince the other half that falling in love with him was a terrific idea. Neither side could be convinced. And it was easy to feel close to him because I couldn't see him. I also couldn't see that he lived, 790 miles away, with the twentysomething-year-old woman he'd been dating. They had absolutely broken up, he said, absolutely, but they were still living together. There were leases and sofas and tables and feelings, he said, "But I wouldn't be talking to you like this if we hadn't broken up, of course."

"Of course," I said. How could he talk to me for so many hours for so many days if they hadn't broken up? I believed him. I believed us both. I had to, to solve the Bolden Offspring Equation correctly.

I made another appointment with the doctor. I told him I knew the end of the rope was very near, but things might be happening. Even now, I'm not sure if I believed myself, if I really believed there was a chance that things would work out between him and me. I am sure that I needed to believe that it had all been worth it, all those years of pain and blood, and so I told myself that this story would have the ending I thought it should have if I could just find some way to wait.

The doctor disappeared behind my chart and made a series of strange, confused sounds before he said, "Okay. Let's try one last thing. Maybe we can buy you some time."

I tried not to hear "one last thing." "Okay," I said. "I'm game."

He suggested a Mirena IUD. "We've seen promising results with endometriosis patients who don't respond to other treatments, since it delivers hormones directly to the site."

He said, "There have also been promising results with fibroids."

He paused. "Of course, your fibroid is very large."

I nodded. "Of course."

"Of course, you have a very aggressive case of endometriosis," he said.

I nodded. "Of course."

"If we can just get you relief long enough for you to have a baby," the doctor said. "Of course, intervention will probably be necessary for you to conceive."

I nodded again. "Of course."

Neither of us said, *If you hurry.* Neither of us said, *If you can.*

For a while, after the Mirena, I was better.

For a little while, I became a new person. A hopeful person, with things to look forward to. Beautiful things. I became a new person who tried to do the kinds of things that a hopeful person with beautiful things to look forward to would do. Cassandra and I walked through the farmers' market on Saturdays. I bought bags of potatoes and bunches of rainbow chard and free-range chicken eggs. I took morning walks through the neighborhood before it gathered its clouds of gnats and heat and humidity. I listened to Beyoncé while putting on my makeup and—terribly, arrhythmically—I tried to dance. On the phone, the man and I talked about *Star Wars* and poems to read at weddings and babies spitting up on sport coats. I imagined mowed lawns and soccer cleats and softball gloves. I imagined myself opening an oven, bending down without pain and straightening up without passing out. I imagined a magazine-perfect roast beef, potatoes swimming in its broth. I imagined a tableclothed table and I sat us in chairs around it. I put two beers and a baby monitor on it, and in the movie I'd made in my mind, we were exhausted but happy. We stayed there, in the house my mind built, and we had everything, anything, we could ever need.

I was a new person. For about two months. At the most.

106

WHILE I WAS DATING MEN AND MAKING EQUATIONS, MY mother would sometimes ask me to consider the validity of a number of arguments. Here is her main argument: that I would be fused to this man for as long as we both lived on the earth and inside of its atmosphere, since I would always be the mother of our biological offspring and he would always be the father of our biological offspring.

"Think about it, Em. Really think," she'd say. "Do you want this person to be part of the rest of your life?"

"I know, and I really am really thinking," I'd say, and then I'd ask her a question, something like, "Do you know how to get the fish smell out of a garbage disposal," so I wouldn't have to know or to really think about it.

A few weeks after the Mirena began to work, I flew home for my father's birthday. I sat at my mother's kitchen table, shaking colored sugar over buttercream-frosted cupcakes.

"You just look so happy," my mother said. We were both smiling in a sugary kind of way, but I looked her in the eye and she looked me in the eye and for a moment something hung between us, some kind of electrical understanding, palpable as heat shimmering above the blacktop in July. I looked away.

"I'm just worried," she said, and when I asked why, my voice was a child's voice. "Because I know why you're happy," she said, "and

I don't want to watch you go through it again." I pushed my teeth against one another until I could feel the pressure in my cheeks. I switched to the blue sparkle sugar, which looked like a glitter of rain.

She wasn't saying and I wasn't saying something we both knew very well: I had given my heart to another man I didn't know very well, if at all. I'd given my heart and hopes to a man I wanted to become a husband, a father. I wanted to believe I knew him. I wanted to think I knew what I wanted, what I was doing. I wanted to think I was thinking this through instead of forcing a stranger into the narrative my body was writing for me.

"I know," I said.

I did not know.

I focused so intensely and intently on finding the right solution for the Bolden Offspring Equation that I never considered the possibility that I'd made a grievous error when I made the equation in the first place. I never considered that perhaps I'd forgotten about the existence and in this case necessity of conditional statements, of hypotheses and conclusions. Or rather, I had forced myself to ignore them. I had built for myself a way of looking at my life that seemed determined upon one fixed ultimate answer.

Take the equation:

I am __ years old. If I date Man __ for __ years before we get married, and if Man __ and I are married for __ years before we produce biological offspring, I will be able to produce a biological offspring before I am age __. Were any of the variables to be filled with zeroes, the equation failed and fell apart; therefore, none of the variables could be zeroes.

I had been thinking of the problem only in terms of the solution. I never considered the possibility that the parts of the equation were wrong, or that they wouldn't fit together, that perhaps I would date but never marry Man __, or perhaps I would date and marry Man __ but never succeed at producing a biological offspring. I never considered the possibility that the existence of the equation itself was wrong, that if I really, deeply thought about it, I might not actually want to date or marry or participate in sexual intercourse with any man so that we could produce a biological offspring. I'd been taught that was what I wanted, and I wanted to be a good student. A good patient. A good girl. I wanted to be good.

If mathematics is "rightly viewed," Bertrand Russell writes, it "possesses not only truth, but supreme beauty—a beauty cold and austere, like that of sculpture, without appeal to any part of our weaker nature, without the gorgeous trappings of painting or music."

Had my high school algebra teacher told us this as a way of telling us that he was not (1) alone, (2) wrong, or (3) all of the above in his assertions about mathematics and beauty, it wouldn't have mattered. We all lived so intensely inside of the limits of our own particular arts and minds and lives that it was often impossible for us to see beauty anywhere and/or everywhere else.

107

IF I AM HONEST, I DIDN'T REALLY THINK OF HAVING A HUSBAND or having a child in anything other than theoretical terms. If I am being more honest, when I did, it terrified me. But I told myself it'd be something that felt right, when I got it, just like it felt right when I got a goldfish even though I was terrified of fish to the point that the presence of an aquarium in the room made me feel hot and dizzy, made me have to leave the room before I threw up or passed out.

The man I'd been talking to moved, so I shared a city with him. And with his girlfriend. She moved in with him and into her own job, where she wore peplum dresses and high heels and presumably never fell down in anyone's driveway.

"I didn't know she was moving," he told me. "I had no idea. I had no idea."

"I don't care if you did." I tried very hard to sound calm and instead just sounded like someone who was trying very hard to be in control. "It's none of my business. Marry her. I don't care." And it wasn't any of my business, but I did care. I couldn't stop searching for her online. All the beautiful things I thought I had to look forward to had vanished, and I told myself that I needed to know why. In all her selfies, she had shining, strong hair and shining, strong teeth, and she seemed the kind of bright and capable woman who will make a very good wife and mother. I watched as her Pinterest boards blossomed with pictures of the perfect picnic and the perfect crib with the perfect Neruda quotes painted on nursery walls. She was building a house in her mind for him, too. She seemed incredibly cruel, though of course she wasn't. She didn't actually know me, if she even knew I existed, and I didn't actually know her.

"Just *stop*," Cassandra said. We were walking through the farmers' market and it was the third time I'd looked at my phone, waiting for a message from the man, scrolling to see if his girlfriend had made another post. I hadn't even looked at the potatoes or chard or chicken eggs of any kind. "You're torturing yourself," she said. But I couldn't stop looking. As if I needed to hurt in a way that I could explain.

Here is how I got a goldfish, even though I was terrified of them to the point of hot and dizzy, to the point of passing out.

It was October and there was a fair. I planned to ride zero rides and eat an entire serving of red velvet funnel cake in order to make myself feel better about, once again, failing to secure a partner who could provide me with offspring. I was not specifically planning to get a goldfish. I was generally unaware that a fair was the kind of place at which one might obtain a goldfish. But one of the first things that I saw that wasn't a terrifying ride or a funnel cake was a table covered in very small glass globes. Around the table stood a circle of people leaning over and making concentration faces, their tongues pink between pink lips, while tossing Ping-Pong balls at the globes. Some used overhand throwing methods. Some used underhand throwing methods. I thought it looked difficult but enjoyable, even though I didn't understand. Then I realized the globes weren't empty. I realized that they were filled with water. Then I noticed that something was *in* the water. Many somethings, in all the many glass globes, and all the somethings were moving. And then the somethings became fish.

I forgot about the red velvet funnel cake and the man and our potential offspring. I forgot about watching the rides for any sights or sounds that might indicate an immediate danger of bodily harm.

I had to have a fish.

Though it wasn't the fish itself I had to have. It wasn't about having, at all. It was about saving. Even though it was October, it was very hot; I had removed my thin cardigan before I even had my hand stamped at the front gates. I couldn't imagine how the fish must've felt, in such small glass globes on such a hot day. How trapped, and also how frightened. To keep swimming and swimming in a circle that small. To be hit, again and again, by Ping-Pong balls.

I gave a man five dollars. I tried both the underhand and overhand throwing methods. I gave a man five more dollars. And then one of my Ping-Pong balls landed in the circle of water at the center of the glass globe.

I had a fish.

After I ate almost an entire way-too-large-for-any-one-human-being serving of red velvet funnel cake, I turned in my ticket, which a man turned into a plastic bag. In its center I saw a bright orange blur of a fish. She swam and shat and looked uncomfortable. I looked, uncomfortably, right back at her. I was terrified but resolute. I wanted to take care of her. I wanted her to be happy and healthy. I waited to see if I would throw up or pass out and when I somehow didn't, I decided to name her Esther Williams, after one of my grandmother's favorite movie stars.

"I want," I told Cassandra, who told me I'd find another man, who told me I'd be okay and watched me eat an entire way-too-large-for-any-one-person serving of red velvet funnel cake without judging me, "to give Esther Williams the best damn life a damn fish could ever dream of having."

In that moment, I felt as much like a mother as I would ever feel.

108

THE MIRENA STOPPED WORKING.
I bled every day for six months.

109

BECAUSE I WORKED AS AN ACADEMIC, I SPENT MY midtwenties through my midthirties moving, preparing to move, or thinking about how I would soon need to move. I moved from college to college, state to state, temporary position to temporary position to, finally, tenure-track position. It's what all my professors and colleagues told me I should want, so I told myself it was what I wanted, too. And there was one big benefit, one thing that I definitely wanted, though I would never admit it to myself: moving made it easier to slip out of people's lives.

I stopped talking on the phone. I took longer and longer to respond to texts until I was hardly responding to them at all. The worse the pain got and the worse I got at dealing with the pain, the more I locked out the world.

This is something I would like to be able to explain, but I can't, not fully. When I try, I say that I only had room for the pain. I say that my friends' lives grew while my life shrank. I say I saw in their lives an opening into the kinds of possibilities that had closed for me, one by one. I say I hurt. I say it hurt, watching them move through the first dates and first kisses and first sleepovers, the meetups for pizza that became wine and nice restaurants that became cohosted cocktail parties in coinhabited apartments, the rings and the mortgages and the birth control pills tossed into the trash can. How they walked into each new stage of adulthood with the expectation that each possibility would just be there, waiting for them. I couldn't see the touchstones in their lives as anything but an illustration of what was missing in mine. Like a camera. Shuttering. I told myself it was the only way to survive.

When Pythagorean mathematicians discovered irrational numbers, they were shocked. They were angry. They balked: the irrational was inelegant, was nothing close to beautiful. And because these numbers were not beautiful, because their very existence created a fault line in the perfection of the world itself, the mathematicians refused to believe in them as true. They couldn't stand the tremors, the way they made their way of viewing the world itself as a beautiful thing shake and shake and shake.

It was almost friendly, the way pain felt familiar, like a sister you have to love because she is your own blood.

Here's how most Saturday nights in my early thirties started: polite-to-the-point-of-silence awkwardly at some faculty friend's party, loosely themed around niche cuisines or experimental craft cocktails flavored with stone fruits and winter produce and herbs. We sat around the table and stared at our drinks to avoid staring at one another, wiping the sweat off our collins glasses and then wiping the sweat off the backs of our necks with our cooled hands. I focused acutely on my own discomfort and on the questions that kept asking themselves: *Can everyone see how much I'm sweating, can everyone tell how much blood I am at this moment losing, what happens if I bleed through all the female hygiene items stuffed in my purse before the middle of this party?*

I started drinking as soon as I got to each party. I grabbed a beer and slid into a corner and snuck a swig—a long swig, a half-the-bottle swig—to make the questions disappear. Then I pregamed with beer at my house, before I even left for the party. I skipped preparty beer and went straight for preparty gin cocktails. I skipped the cocktails and drank the gin straight. Then I skipped the parties and drank the gin straight. I stayed home and in pain and there was always blood, so I'd open a bottle of red wine and pour a glass. I never waited for it to breathe. I sipped. I guzzled. I gulped. I swallowed a Percocet and a Phenergan with a mouthful of red wine. I thought and didn't think about liver damage. I thought and didn't think about my grand-mother, how she said mixing pain pills and liquor would loosen you up, you know, just enough to make the pill work. I sat on my couch and I drank the next glass. The next glass. Then the wine disappeared and I didn't even think about it, how it went down so quickly. I sat on the couch, spinning, and I walked outside to chain-smoke the cigarettes I'd bought for parties. I'd bummed too many from friends.

I was getting to the point of being the girl no one wants to be. I was getting to the point where I no longer wanted to be. I stood on my screened porch and shot cigarette smoke out into the air and then I was crying, I was this thing, this acid-tasting, ruined fruit of a thing saying to herself *oh God oh God*. I thought, *What if I just screamed right now, what if I just opened my mouth and aimed at the moon and just fucking howled, what if I just kept fucking howling until someone in a white coat showed up and took me somewhere where I don't have to be me?* I didn't know how much more I could take. And I didn't know who I could tell that. So I didn't tell anyone. I stayed quiet. I stamped out my cigarette. I weave-walked back into the house and pointedly refused to shower and folded my body in my bed with my heating pad. I stared at the clock. The clock stared back at me. I opened my mouth and I wanted to scream but I didn't. I couldn't. I'd never stop.

It felt, and exactly, like drowning. I felt like I felt at age four, star-ing up at the surface in the bottom of my aunt's pool. I felt like that, like I was surrendering, but I didn't feel the peace. I just kept trying to keep looking up. I just kept trying to breathe.

110

I DON'T REMEMBER WHY CASSANDRA AND I STOPPED BEING friends.

That is, at least, what I want to say.

Or I want to say it's because she found a man who was kind and chopped onions and brought over bottles of very good whiskey, who ate popcorn and M&Ms with us, who Priam trusted enough to let him take him onto the lawn to do whatever he needed to do. I want to say it's because I felt like a third wheel. Because they were part of a couple now and needed friends who were also part of a couple and I couldn't be that friend. I want and don't want to say that every moment between them—every time she reached to hold his hand or he reached to push a strand of hair behind her ear—seemed the most enormous thing, indicative of the fact that they shared the kind of intimacy that led to vows and forevers and white gowns and baby showers, the kind of intimacy I would never—it became more clear, every day—share with another human.

I stopped saying yes when she asked me to come over for dinner and terrible television, to meet her and her boyfriend at the Mellow Mushroom for pizza and those hard apple cider drinks no one else ever ordered. I pretended to be very busy. I pretended to have so very many things to do that I didn't get her texts or emails or Facebook messages until it was too late. Then she had an interview with a school in New Mexico, and then a campus visit—I congratulated her, I was rooting for her, but I was sorry, I couldn't go out to celebrate, it had just been such a long week—and then she had a job. Her boy-friend did, too. I pretended to be very busy until she wrote that she didn't understand what had happened between us. That she missed me. That she was sad that I didn't come to their going-away party. That she just wanted to see me, that one last time. I wrote back that I already missed her terribly. That I would keep missing her terribly.

I meant it.

I wished her every happiness in every world. That was what she deserved. I told her that I hadn't gotten the invitation. I must have missed it. I was just so busy, all the time.

I want to apologize. I want to excuse. I want to say, *Cassandra, I am sorry, I had a nervous breakdown I drank too much I've stopped drink-ing I didn't realize I didn't appreciate you were so good to me, I was this terrible shudder of flesh, as I'm writing this it has been three years and six months since I've seen you, do you remember me, do I want you to remember me, the smoke and the sour and the cereal bowls left stacked in the sink, the coffeepot percolating in perpetuity, I have changed I stopped drinking, forgive me, some days I could not stand and all days I could not stand myself, forgive me, even now I can't stop myself from giving all these excuses.*

There are no reasons. What else can I say? I shuttered my life and I shoved you away.

111

WHEN I WAS THIRTY-TWO, MY MOTHER CAME AND STAYED with me for a reason neither of us particularly wished to recognize, much less verbalize: I could not take care of myself. I could not take care of myself and my cats and my duplex and my students. I could not teach and grade and stop by the BI-LO for milk on the way home. I couldn't sort and separate laundry or hang up the pants to dry or fold the towels once my dryer got finished with them. I could teach. Sort of. Sometimes I sat through the entire class, pain sirening through me.

Sometimes I needed to write something at the board—say, *anaphora* or *homoeoteleuton* or *deus ex machina*—and looked at the three feet between the place where I was sitting and the place where I would have to stand to write on the whiteboard. I'd think to myself, *Nope.* I'd tell my students it wasn't important as I made myself a note: *No h-word on quiz.* I felt guilty. Like a heap of wet leaves instead of the teacher my professors had been, the teacher I imagined I'd once been. I reminded myself that this was ableism and then I felt even more guilty. My mother scooped cat litter and folded towels and fitted sheets and cooked chicken soup and did all the things I no longer had the room to do. All I had room for was the pain. Some nights, I played a game with my mind to make it stop thinking about pain. About guilt. I tried to name an animal for every letter of the alphabet in order—*anteater, beaver, coyote, dog, elephant, fox.*

It never worked.

I had to make a decision. Soon. And I knew what that decision would probably be: a total hysterectomy. I couldn't keep doing this to my mother anymore. Or to my father, who called us at 7:30 every night while he drank Gatorade and recovered from the gym to talk to me and my mother and my cats, who loved him obsessively and rubbed their cheeks against the phone when they heard his voice. I couldn't keep doing this to my mother or my father or my cats or to any of the people I seemed to be letting down in spectacular ways.

But it was hard.

It was hard in the kinds of unspeakable ways that I couldn't put into words then, that instead lived inside of silence. It lived inside of the sound that screamed out of my mouth when I stepped out of the shower and realized I hadn't felt either of my feet step onto the floor. I sat wrapped in a towel on my toilet and started to cry and shut my eyes until I heard my mother run into the bathroom, saying, "Baby, what's wrong? What's wrong?" And I said, "I can't feel my feet." Except I wasn't saying, I wasn't talking, I was sobbing. I was the sound that kept coming and coming from my mouth as my mother pressed my wet face into her shoulder and said, "I know, baby, it's okay, I know."

When the words came to my mouth, there were two of them: *I'm scared.* "I'm scared, I'm scared." I said it over and over. And my mother said, "Me too, baby, I am too." She pulled my body into the crook of her body and we rocked. We rocked until I wasn't screaming or sobbing, I was just exhausted and wet and cold and shivering in my towel, sitting on the toilet. My mother tore off a wad of toilet paper and handed it to me to blow my nose. Then she tore off a wad of toilet paper and blew her nose. We sat there and breathed for a minute. And then I realized I was still breathing. I could feel that. I was still alive. I wiped my eyes. "I'm so sorry," I said.

"Peanut, if I could take this away from you," my mother said, "I'd do it in a heartbeat. But I can't. So we'll figure it out." She put her hand on my knee, like she always did when I was in pain, like she always did in the doctor's office when we faced a moment in which my body and the things it did became inexplicable. "We'll figure it out."

I told myself that when I was sick, my parents were the only people I let in because they had to love me just because they were my parents and I was their child. This was wrong, and I knew it. No matter how much I broke, I knew that they would still choose to love me. I knew they had the choice. I knew what kind of people they were. I knew what choice they would make.

112

IN THE SIXTH MONTH OF BLEEDING, AFTER MY MOTHER HAD gone home, I had to decide if I was going to let my body stop me from traveling to a writer's conference to give a talk about writing from memory. I decided to cancel. Then I decided to go. I decided I was sick of it holding me back. The pain and the numbness. The bleeding.

My mother sent a text: *Have you packed yet? Don't wait until the last minute, you'll forget something. By the way I am watching Jack.* My cousin Jessica's son. He'd become her surrogate grandchild, which made me feel a kind of fury too sad and complicated to analyze or explain, and so I just told myself that I was at peace with it. I told myself that I was happy, for my mother. My cousin had given her what I cannot.

Jack wanted to see a picture of my fish, the next text said, so I stood in front of her tank, clicking photos with my cell phone while she bubbled and swished from one side to the other. Some of the photos were orange blurs, some just the wash of a fin through water. In most of the photos, she looked elongated, eyeless and mouthless, mutated by the curved plastic of the tank. I got one photo of an almost-right almost-whole fish, finally, and sent it to my mother, to my cousin's son.

Tell Jack she was too busy dancing for me to get a good picture, I texted her.

You are so good with kids, she texted back.

Yes, I thought. *I'm good with kids.* I thought, *I would've made a good mother.* I thought, *But could I have been a good mother longer than the time it took to send this text?*

When my mother had told me over the phone that my cousin Jessica was pregnant, I asked her the questions people are expected to ask when they find out that another person is pregnant. These questions include but are not limited to: *How far along is she, what's her due date, how is she feeling, is it a boy or a girl, when will she find out if it is a boy or a girl?* I fought against crying. I won until I hung up the phone. Then I began chanting-sobbing-saying *it's not fair it's not fair.* I threw a Moleskine notebook (1) against the wall and (2) as hard as I could, which was not very hard but was still enough to leave a mark. I felt both satisfied and embarrassed.

113

WHILE I ATTENDED CATHOLIC SCHOOL, I WAS PERIODICALLY required to receive the holy Sacrament of Reconciliation. I stood in a line with the other Roman Catholic students, then went into a room where I may or may not have been able to see the priest, depending upon the absence or presence of a screen. I told the priest and God that I wished to be blessed, that I had sinned. I told them how long it'd been since I'd received the holy Sacrament of Reconciliation. I told them that I was heartily sorry for my sins.

One sin for which I was heartily sorry every single time: being jealous of my cousin Jessica. She had a Barbie Dreamhouse, a new Barbie car and not a hand-me-down Barbie car that reeked of every cigarette ever secretly smoked in our aunt's garage, a better bike, a Lite Brite that she didn't even use. She had a better head of better hair, stone-dark brown eyes better than my whiskey-weak brown eyes, boyfriends who gave her genuine leather shoes and/or sterling silver jewelry, and the instinct for wearing exactly enough blush.

It's still true that I am jealous of my cousin Jessica today, though I no longer go to confession, which may or may not be why it is still true today.

I wonder now if my problem with algebra was ultimately a problem of solvability. There was something beautiful—my teacher was right—about the mystery, the letters and symbols that could, in their equations, mean or come to mean anything. It was a different thing that frightened me: the idea that there was always an answer there, waiting, always one single true answer I'd be forced to find if I did my calculations correctly. It was the idea that that single true answer wouldn't be the answer I had assumed. I thought my answer was to get married and have a baby. Without that answer, how could I justify it? The hours I spent inside of a body that seemed so intent on producing nothing but pain? I thought there had to be a viable explanation, a point in time from which I could look backward and say, *This was all worth it, because I am now here, because this child also is now here.* Without that point, without that answer, where would I be, and how would I be able to look back over all the wheres and the whos I had been?

As I drove to the airport to catch a plane for the conference, I kept feeling very proud of myself for keeping Esther Williams the fairground fish alive for a year. I also began to worry. That one of my cats would figure out, finally, some way to open the aquarium and eat the fish inside. That she wouldn't like her three-day vacation feeder, or that she wouldn't find it, or that she'd forget how to eat from it, though she had seemed to enjoy her previous experiences with it as much as a fish can seem to enjoy anything. I worried that somehow, some way, I had cursed her, by thinking so much and so proudly about having kept her alive for so long.

114

A FRIEND AND I SHARED A ROOM AT THE CONFERENCE. FROM our separate beds in our together hotel room, we talked about our postsexual lives. We talked about relief. We said we missed the companionship of romantic relationships, the camaraderie. We missed the good-morning coffee, the spiked good-night decaf. We missed the romance, of course, but that's like missing the fjords, or missing the midnight sunset, or missing our long and celebrated Broadway careers, or any of the thousand other nouns and verbs we never had. We did not miss the pressure, metaphorical or literal, of our sexual lives. And I was happy talking, happy chatting, happy offering halves of Diet Cokes and chocolate walnut cookies. I was happy watching television when a commercial for *Les Misérables* came on. Then I was happy-singing and she was happy-singing about stars, there, out in the darkness. It was her favorite song from *Les Mis*, she said, her favorite favorite one, and because I was happy I said it was mine too, and I happy-sang and she happy-sang about stars and the night.

I want this story to be better orchestrated. I want there to be crescendo and crash, a moment when revelation shatters my soul like a glass that can't stand up to the high notes. But there are no high notes. There's no buildup and no crash. There was no eureka, no one moment when I knew, when I made my decision. There was instead a slow recognition not of what I no longer had but what I'd never had in the first place, an acknowledgment that all the things I felt slipping away from my grasp were never in my grasp. There is no bang nor whimper. There is instead my face in the mirror watching its mouth open, calmly quiet, around the word *enough*.

"Stars" is, of course, not my favorite favorite, or even my favorite, song from *Les Mis*. My favorite song, my favorite favorite, is and always has been "I Dreamed a Dream," which Fantine sings from the floor of the stage in a tattered dress patterned with the same Laura Ashley roses as my childhood bedspread. She sings about a time when world and song were thrilling, a time before things went wrong. It seemed so true, even when I was a child. It always seemed as if things, whatever things were, had already gone or soon would go wrong.

When I got home from the conference, I saw her: a sad, curled comma of a fish, floating.

WITHOUT THE GORGEOUS TRAPPINGS

115

HERE ARE THE ANSWERS TO SOME OF THE QUESTIONS YOU may want to ask when you hear that I had a total hysterectomy at the age of thirty-three.

I am the mother of zero biological offspring. No, the doctor did not harvest my eggs. Yes, he removed my ovaries. He also incinerated them in some kind of medical fire. No, I have absolutely no idea how that works. I do, however, know that this means I will never be the mother of biological offspring.

Yes, I did want to have biological offspring. I was not specific with regard to number except that I wanted a number of biological offspring greater than zero, which is the number of biological offspring I had, currently have, or will in the future have.

The technical term for the operation I had is *total hysterectomy with a bilateral salpingo-oophorectomy*. Said surgery entails the following: the complete removal of the uterus, fallopian tubes, ovaries, and cervix from a female human being's body.

According to the websites of various medical organizations (including but not limited to the Mayo Clinic and WebMD), the possible risks of a total hysterectomy include: the formation of adhesions, hemorrhage, bowel obstruction, vaginal prolapse, and urinary incontinence. Possible aftereffects include: premature menopause, a reliance on hormone therapy, osteoporosis, increased concentration, improved job performance, improved interpersonal relationships, and the ability to wear white pants, skirts, and undergarments. What these sites fail to mention as a side and/or aftereffect: it is difficult, if not impossible, to openly discuss this operation and/or its aftereffects. Even in the most technical of terms.

I wanted to have biological children, I guess. I also wanted my parents to have biological grandchildren. I have no brothers or sisters. I am my parents' sole offspring.

Yes, I should have waited longer.
Yes, I should not have waited so long.

I look both exactly like my mother and exactly like my father, depending on (1) whom I'm sitting next to and (2) whom you ask. I have brown hair and brown eyes; my father has brown hair and brown eyes too, and my mother has brown hair and green eyes. As a child, I once asked her when she was going to get her eyes fixed to match my father's and mine. I never really imagined what my offspring would look like, but I did vaguely assume: A human body. Brown eyes. Brown hair. I never considered a father's genetics in my vague assumptions, which says a lot about how I thought about that.

I also never thought about what I wanted my theoretical biological offspring to call me. I only knew that I did not want them to call me *mommy*, which is a word I dislike as a noun, adjective, and verb.

I did think about what my theoretical offspring would call my father and my mother: Dwight and Mamie, respectively.

116

ACCORDING TO THE MAYO CLINIC, "THE EXACT CAUSE OF endometriosis is not certain." The Mayo Clinic offers no opinion as to whether or not endometriosis may be a genetic disease and/or condition. The physicians I saw also stated that they didn't know if endometriosis was genetic, though some said perhaps, it could be, they didn't know, don't quote them on it, okay.

A physician who thinks that endometriosis is, perhaps, genetic might also think that I inherited endometriosis from my mother, who herself suffered from the same Disease and Condition. In fact, I exist solely because my mother took Human Chorionic Gonadotropin (hCG), which, according to the Mayo Clinic, is a fertility drug "used to mature the eggs and trigger their release at the time of ovulation." My mother actually took hCG in order to lose weight. The maturing and triggering of eggs was merely a side effect, as was the person made from one of these eggs: me.

Here is how my mother discovered that she and my father had created a person: when she had lost nearly forty pounds of weight, she put some nice winter-white pants on layaway at Parisian department store. After she received her paycheck, she paid for her pants and took them home and tried them on in her bathroom. She could not button her pants. Were my mother a cartoon character, at this moment a thought bubble would've appeared above her head with a question mark floating inside of it. This was the moment she realized that an offspring might be growing inside of her body.

•

During her diet, my mother also ate six apples and drank two gallons of water every day. The Mayo Clinic does not indicate if apples or water are effective fertility treatments.

Though my mother wanted to produce multiple offspring, the Diseases and Conditions of her reproductive system rendered her infertile. She was just very lucky to happen upon a method for weight loss that incidentally aided in fertility. This is the type of coincidence that she attributes to fate or to God.

I was not lucky in the way that my mother was lucky. I'm not sure if my lack of luck relates to fate or to God. I am not sure if I can entirely believe in the ideas of luck, fate, or God, at least in the benevolent sense.

Sometimes I try to say *I am an only child* and instead say *I am only a child*. This both is and is not accurate.

117

A FEW MONTHS BEFORE MY HYSTERECTOMY, I LOOKED AS though I was pregnant. I realized this when I could not zip up the jeans I had finally lost just enough weight to wear, and then I could not zip up the jeans I was wearing just fine after I'd gained weight. I put on a loose dress and made an appointment with a physician.

I knew I couldn't be actually pregnant because I hadn't engaged in sexual intercourse during the luteal phase of my menstrual cycle. In fact, I hadn't even attempted sexual intercourse in well over a year, and even then it had been unsuccessful. I still worried. I still asked myself, *What if when you were very, very drunk you engaged in sexual intercourse and then forgot about it?* Then I remembered that I had in fact not been very, very drunk for well over a year. I had only been approximately drunk, and only once, while in my own pajamas in my own house with my own bottle of pink wine, watching *Dateline* and not engaging in sexual intercourse with anyone or anything.

The fact that I had not engaged in sexual intercourse or been very, very drunk over approximately the same stretch of time is not a coincidence.

Yes, of course, I have cats.

I have two female cats, Gertrude Stein and Alice B. Toklas.

Neither have had sexual partners since they became my cats. This is because they live exclusively inside of my house, where they lick their legs and watch me when I watch *Dateline* and throw Moleskine notebooks against the wall.

My female cats have not had, do not currently have, and will not in the future have biological offspring. This is because my female cats were spayed, so all three of us have had total hysterectomies.

I did not inform the fertility specialist that I focused on getting degrees in my early twenties because degrees interested me and sexual intercourse did not. I assumed that my lack of interest in sexual intercourse was merely a symptom that would go away if I found the right treatment for my Diseases and Conditions.

I first considered the possibility of a hysterectomy when the Diseases and Conditions affecting my reproductive system became so severe that I had trouble feeding my cats, changing their litter boxes, and attempting to trim their fingernails with pet-safe claw clippers. Also, I wasn't sure how much longer I could keep my reproductive organs and keep working, which meant that I wasn't sure how much longer I could afford to keep my cats.

I am aware that calling my cats' claws fingernails makes me sound crazy because my mother once said, "Don't call your cats' claws fingernails. It makes you sound crazy."

118

I FIRST HEARD THE WORD *ASEXUALITY* IN 2013 WHEN A student said to me, "I am asexual and no one understands."

I nodded.

I said, "I understand." And I did understand, though I didn't fully know it or know why. I waited until I got home to google *asexuality*. I was afraid to use my computer at work. I don't know if I was afraid of someone finding out that I suspected I might be asexual or if I was afraid of myself finding out that I suspected I might be asexual.

I learned from Wikipedia that an asexual is someone who experiences a "lack of sexual attraction to others, or low or absent interest in or desire for sexual activity." I learned from the Asexual Visibility and Education Network that an asexual is "someone who does not experience sexual attraction." Asexuality, I read, is not a choice but a sexual orientation.

I read both definitions again. I sat still. I looked at the computer screen for a little while, thinking *what*. Just like that, with no question mark.

There weren't any more questions.

119

THE LAST TIME I REMEMBER USING THE ADJECTIVE *SEXY* IN reference to myself was approximately seven hours after my hysterectomy. I hadn't slept. There was blood and pain. I felt better than I had in at least ten years. The nurse handed me a pair of paper underwear that were more like loose, thin shorts than underwear. I said, "Oh, these are sexy." And she said, "Victoria's real secret."

"It isn't that *I* don't find you sexually attractive," a man I was dating once said. "It's that *you* aren't sexually attractive. I'm sorry. It's true. You are many things, but you are not sexy."

It was a Saturday near the end of the third month in which we had occasionally shared beds. I did not respond.

On Monday, I decided to approach the problem academically. I asked myself two questions: (1) *What is sexually attractive*, and (2) *How can I become sexually attractive?* A quick Google search delivered photographs of pink, mostly nude women. My stomach quivered. And it wasn't an excited quiver but an I-am-very-nauseated quiver, the same quiver I felt when I found a 1950s recipe for Jell-O with cubes of ham inside. I asked myself, *Why this kind of quivering, the Jell-O ham quivering?*

I clicked on a photo of Bettie Page, all leopard and breast and cropped bangs. If she quivered, she didn't show it. She seemed empowered beyond nausea, with her lipstick and her whip.

On Tuesday, I shivered in a silver salon chair, a black drape tied around my neck in a way that, had I been Bettie Page, might've been sexy. "Bangs," I said. "Schoolgirl style." With my index finger, I drew a line barely above my eyebrows, the way villains draw lines across their throats. You're dead.

Later, I met the man I was dating for dinner. I'd already had a glass of loosen-up wine. I'd already started and stopped myself from asking, a hundred times: *Why is schoolgirl style a sexy style? How long have I carried this idea within me, how did I let it fall so easily out of my lips and then just leave it there, quivering?*

"So you got bangs," he said, plain as a napkin. I knew then. I should've left him. But I told myself to hold on. If I found the right doctor, I could find the right cure. I could find some way to be attractive. To feel attraction. I told myself I deserved it, his every single word.

120

THERE ARE, OF COURSE, SYNONYMS FOR THE WORD *ASEXUAL*, all of which hit a different note.

There's *celibacy*, the choice to not have sex.

There's *low sex drive*, a term that implies its opposite—*high sex drive*—and therefore describes desire as an impulse that may wane but can wax again.

There's *frigidity*, a word that's also a punishment. A slur that freezes women into the dangerous implication that if a woman denies a man sex, that woman is doing something wrong—or that there is something wrong with her.

There's *hypoactive sexual desire disorder* (HSDD), also known as *inhibited sexual desire* (ISD). Both, according to the *Diagnostic and Statistical Manual of Mental Disorders*, are mental illnesses. According to the Mayo Clinic, they are physical and/or mental illnesses.

Here is a confession: the paper hospital underwear were fantastic.

They were so fantastic that I spent a considerable amount of time searching for terms like *paper underwear* and *postsurgical underpants* on Google and Amazon. I never received an accurate result. I still wish that I had.

•

On the front page of the Asexual Visibility and Education Network's website, there used to be the following caveat to the very concept of asexuality:

> **Note**: People do not need sexual arousal
> to be healthy, but in a minority of cases
> a lack of arousal can be the symptom of
> a more serious medical condition. If you
> do not experience sexual arousal or if
> you suddenly lose interest in sex you
> should probably check with a doctor just
> to be safe.

The caveat has since been deleted. Still I sometimes feel it, like a ghost, whispering: *What does that even* mean?

121

I ASKED MY PARENTS IF THEY WERE OKAY WITH MY HAVING A hysterectomy without first having a husband and/or my own biological offspring. It was a very strange conversation to have, a *hey do you mind if your genetic line ends with me because I failed to produce a biological offspring* kind of conversation. Though medical websites offer advice for talking to one's doctor about a hysterectomy, I could find no advice for talking to one's parents about the termination of their genetic line.

It is entirely possible that the *Diagnostic and Statistical Manual of Mental Disorders* and the Mayo Clinic and the Asexual Visibility and Education Network and the man I once dated are all correct, when it comes to me, that asexuality may be related to my medical history. When I started my period, I started experiencing symptoms of polycystic ovary syndrome, which caused my ovaries to make more androgens than they're supposed to make. This made my female body trend slightly more toward the male, sprouting facial hair and body hair along with my zits. I also started experiencing symptoms of endometriosis, including cramps and bleeding that soon became so paralyzingly bad that I was faced with a choice: take hormones to prevent ovulation and menstruation or fail out of school before I finished eighth grade.

This, of course, was not a choice.

I wonder: How many things are?

I wonder: Who am I betraying by voicing these questions? And if I stay silent, who will I betray?

122

I LIED WHEN I SAID THAT I ASKED BOTH MY FATHER AND MY mother if they were okay with my hysterectomy. I know and with certainty that I asked my mother. It was one of those conversations that human beings have with one another in which they (1) cry and (2) hold one another, and (3) sort of rock back and forth. My mother called me baby and in the voice with all the sadnesses in it and I cried in that strange voiceless way.

I do not remember with certainty if I asked my father.

If I didn't ask my father, it wasn't because I'm not close enough to him to ask that kind of question. It wasn't because my father is a male human being and wouldn't understand, because even though he is a male human being, he would very much understand. It was probably because when I think of my father, I think of being a little girl, when he read me stories about Muppets and bears on great adventures and pollen-yellow-haired girls who disagreed with the bears' household decisions, and that made me feel so happy and sad that I couldn't ask him if it was okay that I'd never have an offspring to whom he could read those same stories.

I told very few people that I was going to have a hysterectomy: My friend Deena. My conference friend. My department chair and my departmental secretary, because I had to pull out of teaching a summer course and felt they needed an adequate explanation. My mother told a few family members, but, for the most part, I kept the operation a secret. A silence. I do and I don't know why. There was shame. There was embarrassment. There was the shuddering feeling of failure, the back-of-my-Catholic-schoolgirl-mind flutter of an awareness of sin. There were so many questions I expected people to ask: *Why? How are you? Have you exhausted all other options? Why did you wait so long? Why don't you wait a little longer? Are you sure about this?* And if I wasn't asked, I could pretend I knew the answers. I could pretend that there were answers. I could pretend that I believed there was ultimately anything in and about this world that wasn't just another question.

I haven't received the holy Sacrament of Reconciliation since I received the holy Sacrament of Confirmation. Should I in the future receive the holy Sacrament of Reconciliation, I'd say to the priest and to God, by way of the priest, *Forgive me, Father, for I have sinned.* I'd lie and say, *I do not remember the date of my last good confession.* I'd say, *I am heartily sorry for my sins, Father, I would rather run away than talk through all the difficult things, Father, I am jealous of my cousin Jessica, for You have given unto her so many gifts, can You not see that my arms are empty and my womb is missing?*

I'd say, *Father, I might've lied about not remembering the date of my last good confession.*

I'd say, *I am heartily sorry for these and all the sins of my past life.*

123

THE LAST TIME I DYED MY HAIR, I USED THE JOLEN CREME Bleach I'd bought to bleach the dark stripe of hair that moved in above my lip when my natural estrogen moved out. For months, I'd scrolled through a thousand Pinterest photos of a thousand heads dyed every imaginable color. It was as if the world had awakened into a new and neon future and, once again, I'd left myself behind. I wanted to be awakened. I wanted to see myself in color, somehow.

In the bathroom, I listened to Tori Amos thunder down the piano, trembling between sadness and fury. I put my hair in a bun and pulled a thick set of strands from the bottom. I coated them in bleach, acrid and gritty. Long before I'd begun to exist in my body, to walk and talk and look at bodies and think, *There's something I'm missing, something I just can't see*, Alfred Kinsey and his colleagues began to realize that sometimes the reason why you can't find yourself on a spectrum is because you exist in a place outside of that spectrum. A zero on the Kinsey Scale indicated absolute heterosexuality; a six indicated the same about homosexuality. But there's a value missing from the scale, a value that Kinsey nonetheless noticed and determined was important enough to note in both *Sexual Behavior in the Human Male* and *Sexual Behavior in the Human Female*: X. An absence of attraction.

I thought that when I had a hysterectomy, I'd be cured. I thought I'd find what was missing, that I'd see what I just couldn't see. I told myself the pain was holding me back from feeling attraction; I never considered that not feeling attraction might instead be an integral part of me. My hysterectomy wasn't the cure I wanted to find. I didn't gain the ability to feel and understand attraction, but I did gain the ability to understand at least one small part of myself. I'd sought relationships because I wanted to have a child; when that factor disappeared, the equation collapsed, which was its own solution. I'd discovered that, in my case, an X was just an X. The absence of attraction was its own presence.

I still don't know how to talk about myself, sexually. I don't know if that sentence should read, "I don't know how to talk about myself, sexually" or "I don't know how to talk about my sexuality." I still don't know what terms to use, if there are terms to use, if terms do anything other than offer a name for the peculiar difficulties of living inside a human body. And so with one friend, I use the word *celibate*. With another, I use the term *postsexual*. I use it in a sentence. I say, "If I wasn't *postsexual*, I totally would have flirted with him." She uses it in a sentence back: "Well, when you stop being *postsexual* and start being *sexual-sexual*, you can flirt with him." She changes the definition, and I want to change it back, to tell her that there wasn't a before and there probably won't be an again, but it's too clumsy and bothersome a thing to pass over the tongue.

With my mother, I am too embarrassed to use terms, so I say, "Maybe I should have been a nun." With a physician, I say, "I have not engaged in sexual intercourse for a very long time." She says, "Like, several months?" I say, "No, like several years." She checks a box on her chart. I know there is a word there. I know she is using that word to define me.

I don't ask her what it is.

With myself, I say *asexual*. Then I stop. And then I wonder: *Is this my sexuality or is it a medical condition, where do the body and the self meet and where do the body and the self part, what parts of the self are the body, where do I look for definition?* I take a deep breath. I sit for a moment. I say it to myself again. *Asexual.*

I do not argue.

I washed out the bleach and then carefully, latex-gloved, spread pink dye over the place where color had once been. After I'd washed out the dye, pink remained. I picked up a hand mirror so I could see what others saw when I walked away: a solid sheet of brown. I put my hair in a ponytail and aimed the mirror just so, again. I saw it: a hot little ribbon of pink. A mark of identity that, even when hidden, remained ready to do what I and my words could not do. To admit. To declare. To scream.

My parents asked me to go to mass with them after my hysterectomy, so I went to mass. I made the sign of the cross. I genuflected. I sat between them in a pew. I watched and stood and sat and kneeled. I followed along in the missalette. When the parishioners spoke, I stayed silent.

The priest said it was important to keep the rituals of the church, to prepare our bodies to receive Communion through hours of fasting before mass. And it was important to demonstrate those rituals for our children, to practice them as a family. He spoke of the absolute importance of family, the necessity of having children and passing on the faith to them. "The way to salvation," he said, "is through family." I stayed sitting in the pew between my parents, then I sat in the back seat of their car, then I sat with them in a booth in a Mexican restaurant, and it wasn't until I was back in my own home and in my own shower with the water running that my body finally folded. I sat on the bathtub floor and cried.

THE SONG THAT HAS NO END

124

Two days after my hysterectomy, I held a nurse's hand and walked out of the hospital and to my mother's car.

"Is she supposed to be walking? Aren't you supposed to use a wheelchair?" I heard the false calm in my mother's voice.

The nurse answered her questions: yes and no, respectively. And so I walked out of hospital, carrying on my own two feet a body that required an instruction manual. Everything felt terribly specific and confusing. There were pills rainbowed across a pill case, each with its own date and time. There were specific instructions regarding underwear. Schedules for bandages. Schedules for slowly increasing physical activity. Cups to catch and measure my urine for signs of urinary retention and infection, as my catheter had been removed too soon. Hormone pills and patches that looked like Nicoderm, sticky with estrogen, which had to be carefully removed and disposed of, as they can cause female characteristics in men. I imagined a man slapping it onto his bicep in the fever of a cigarette craving and growing instant Dolly Parton boobs.

The day after I got home from the hospital, I noticed a gray hair settled in the center of my right eyebrow. "This soon?" I asked it. Before it could answer, I'd plucked it out.

•

I skipped the story of my hysterectomy itself because it doesn't feel like my story. Perhaps this is because it doesn't feel like a story at all. It feels more like a supposition. A presumption. A small series of facts shored up by a larger series of conjectures. Over and over, I shift and shape the details. I ask my mother what she saw and heard. I ask my father what he saw and heard. I ask new doctors, who refuse to comment or speculate. They are afraid of lawsuits and sometimes they admit that. I reshift, reshape. I try to make sense of what I know and don't know. But what I know and don't know resist sense. What I know and don't know struggle against any sense of structure. I can't piece together a cohesive narrative of what has happened to and inside my own body.

Here are the parts of the story I know.

My hysterectomy was scheduled for 10:30 in the morning. I was called into the presurgical holding area. I was given a thin hospital gown, my final pregnancy test, and permission to leave my socks on my feet. I removed all my earrings and swore I had no additional piercings. I lay in the bed as a nurse tried and failed and tried again to find a good vein for my IV. I tried to watch the television. I tried to focus on a commercial for the remake of *The Texas Chainsaw Massacre*, on the engine sound of the blade revving up. I tried not to cry. I cried.

"I'm sorry," I told the nurse. "I'm so sorry."

She patted the spot on my hand that she'd been thumping with her middle finger. "I'm going to give you a minute to rest. I'll give you something for your nerves when we get this IV started."

I know that I waited, and then I waited. I know that the first nurse made good on her promise to give me something for my nerves. It wasn't good enough. By the time I was wheeled back to the operating room, I'd been in the presurgical area for over five hours. I'd seen two shifts of nurses, two shifts of anesthesiologists and their teams. My father had paced the hallway floor approximately seventeen times. My mother had sighed "Jesus, Mary, and Joseph" approximately twenty times. The surgeon had one surgery scheduled before mine, and it was a long and difficult operation.

My parents and I talked over our options in the long, bright breaks between nurse check-ins. Should we go home? Should we ask if the surgeon could wait until the next day, until he'd had sleep and coffee and a good solid meal with vegetables and protein? We never asked the nurses these questions because we knew that there weren't answers. We knew that there weren't options. And so, finally, a nurse took the glasses off my face and handed them to my mother.

My parents told me they loved me and kissed me on the forehead while the nurses pulled up the gates on the sides of my hospital bed. They pushed me through rooms and hallways and doors that, without my glasses, seemed like great white blurs. We rushed to the wing in which the hospital kept its da Vinci system, a robot designed for minimally invasive surgery. Even without my glasses I could see that the wing was still very much under construction, with plastic sheets draped over unfinished spaces, CAUTION and CONSTRUCTION signs hung like strange windows. The robot itself looked like a Transformer gone wrong and I remember asking if they were going to introduce us, me and this machine to which I was entrusting my life.

I know that the surgery was supposed to last four hours, three and a half hours at the absolute least. It was going to take time, the surgeon had said. Time and care. From my past surgical records, he knew that endometriosis implants had sunk deep in my peritoneum, hiding in pockets of tissue. It would take a lot of time to dig that endometriosis out. It would take a lot of time to find and excise every growth, every cyst, every remnant of ovarian tissue and uterosacral ligament.

"Most doctors are afraid to go to this extent," he said at my presurgical consultation, "but I'm not. I always take my time. I always get it done."

I entered the operating room four hours and eight minutes after I was scheduled to.

The surgery lasted an hour and forty-nine minutes, at the absolute max.

The gynecologist I normally saw did not perform my hysterectomy. This is because he was just a normal gynecologist and, he said, I needed an expert. I needed someone who was used to long and extensive surgeries, who was deliberate and accurate and accustomed to searching a woman's pelvis for every small sign of every small thing that shouldn't be in her pelvis. This was especially important when it came to detecting endometriosis. When filled with blood vessels, lesions can be the same pink or red as surrounding tissue. They can also be clear, like tiny blisters. And so the gynecologist referred me to an oncologist who operated in a hospital an hour's drive away.

I saw the oncologist once before my surgery. He reviewed my patient history and performed a physical exam, during which he noted that my uterus was so stuck down with adhesions as to be immobile. "At this point the patient is here," he writes in his notes on that visit, "because she desires definitive therapy." He writes that he spoke with me about freezing my eggs and other fertility options. I am, he writes, uninterested in these.

The fertility options offered by the surgeon were extremely expensive. According to Circle Surrogacy, a Boston-based surrogacy agency, for a U.S. resident who has frozen her own eggs or embryos and just needs a surrogate, the cost is $148,750. If that U.S. resident also requires donor eggs, the price jumps to $172,250. Those prices only cover one round of IVF; most women go through multiple rounds before a pregnancy is successful. According to WebMD, women under the age of thirty-five have only a 37.6 percent chance of successful conception and pregnancy through IVF—if they use their own eggs. In an interview with NPR, University of Southern California fertility specialist Richard Paulson describes the financial toll that IVF can take:

> Many women will have to undergo the procedure more than once. It cost about $10,000 to harvest eggs from the ovaries, after a woman has taken medications for several weeks to stimulate egg production. Then the eggs need to be frozen and stored, at a cost of about $500 a year. Each time eggs are thawed, fertilized and transferred to the uterus with IVF it costs about $5,000.

One of the drugs used to improve egg production in IVF cycles: Lupron.

I don't actually know if the oncologist actually performed my surgery. My operative reports don't know, either. It took six months—and several repeated requests—for a primary care physician to obtain my records. Or, rather, to obtain *some* of my records: the pathologist's report and a partial operative report. The latter was dictated by the surgeon's primary resident the night after my surgery. It had been edited twice. The second edit took place after complications sent me to the emergency room twice.

In his notes from my preoperative assessment, the oncologist omits one very important point: The fertility treatments I was offered and refused did not entirely relate to my own fertility. They were also about the fertility of others. They were about harvesting my own eggs, but by this, the doctor did not mean that I would be the one who used them. I would be the one who sold them, presumably to his patients.

Here is what I know from the operative report: The surgeon was present and in scrubs for the entirety of the operation. However, the operative report avoids pronouns, making the question of who, exactly, performed each part of the surgery even more of a question. So does the lack of detail in the report.

The surgical report is clear about the presence of endometrial implants in my abdomen. At one point, the Description of Operation states that there was "evidence of endometriosis in her posterior cul-de-sac." This is followed directly by this sentence: "At this time, a 1-cm supraumbilical incision was made for the camera port and an additional 3 accessory ports were placed in the usual fashion for robotic surgery." Between these two sentences, there is no description of a careful search for endometriosis, nor of the specific endometrial implants he located and recognized.

There is also no description of the surgeon excising the endometrial implants he located and recognized.

There is no description because he did not excise these endometrial implants.

Therefore, the endometrial implants are still present in my abdomen.

125

On the day of my presurgical testing, I'd started out on my hour-long drive with over twenty minutes to spare. Those twenty minutes were taken up traveling one block on DeRenne Avenue. I passed the sign for Habersham Street, which seemed like an unfair joke. I looked at my GPS, which told another unfair joke: I was going to be late. I called the number on the forms I'd filled out for the hospital, apologized for calling, and told them I was stuck in traffic before apologizing again. I hung up. I started yelling—at the traffic lights, the cars in front of me, the city graying around me, an ambulance, all the moss in the trees. I was both appalled and impressed with myself.

When I made it, finally, to the hospital, a nurse handed me a laminated card with a list of various medical conditions. She told me to tell her which of the conditions I had. I started my recitation: GERD, IBS, stomach problems, bladder problems, bowel problems, frequent falls. Neither of us knew how to classify dysautonomia, or whatever it was that made my legs and arms numb. I watched the glass fishbowl on her desk, with a halfway-floating plastic plant halfway-nestled in Technicolor gravel. At first, I didn't see the fish. Then he halfway-floated toward me and to the surface. He was a black betta and he was clearly almost dead. The water fanned his fins out behind him in a motion that seemed beyond his volition. His front fins wiggled a little and I felt a little better. Then the fins went unmistakably still.

The nurse left to photocopy my preop instructions and the fish floated, limp-lying, up to the top of the bowl. Panic churned my stomach. I got close-but-not-too-close to the bowl and tapped the glass. He didn't move, so the panic moved to my throat. *This is a bad sign*, I thought. *This is a very bad sign.*

I composed myself enough to compose a text message: *I SWEAR TO GOD I AM SITTING IN THE NURSE'S OFFICE DURING PRESURGICAL TESTING AND HER FUCKING FISH JUST FUCKING DIED*, in all caps, just like that. I sent it to Deena.

Fish actually LOVE to die, Deena wrote back. *Your fairground goldfish stayed alive for a year because it was a freak.*

The nurse returned with prescriptions and two pages' worth of instructions for a three-day-long bowel prep. "We want to be as careful as possible, given your previous bowel puncture," she said.

"I think your fish is dead," I said.

She said "really" but seemed unconcerned. "Surely he's not dead. I'm borrowing this office. I don't want to have to say *sorry, your fish died on my watch*." She hit the bowl with her pen and he moved a little. We were both relieved, and the relief gave us room to finish my paperwork.

"Do you have a religious preference?"

I sat with the question for a moment, watching the fish kind-of-float. He didn't offer suggestions. "Roman Catholic," I mumbled.

"Sorry," the nurse said. I heard it as a statement and not a question. Then I realized she hadn't understood.

"Roman Catholic," I said, enunciating each syllable. "I am Roman Catholic." And then the fish fell against the side of the bowl.

"Look at that," the nurse said. "He's all fallen over, isn't he?" She tapped the bowl. He didn't move. "Something's not right," she said.

I agreed.

126

I HAD THIS RITUAL WITH ONE OF MY CATS—OR, RATHER, one of my cats had this ritual with me. Every morning, afternoon, and night, my cat walked with me into my home office, which is where I kept the goldfish I'd won at the fair. She watched as I flipped up the Open tab on the bottle of fish food and obtained approximately one flake of food for every approximate inch of fish. She then watched as I opened the top of the tank and sprinkled approximately three of the aforementioned flakes on the surface of the water. My cat watched, blinking, as my approximately three-inch-long fish swam to the surface, moving her fish lips together and apart, calm in the safety of her tank.

I don't actually know if my fish was female. I just assumed.

Now that the fish is dead, my cat still keeps the ritual. She stands in the hallway each evening, waiting for me, then walks into my home office. She expects me to follow. She meows into the doorframe. She looks, again and again, to the blank space on the top of my file cabinet where the fish tank should still be. She tilts her head, always to the right. If she were a cartoon character and not an actual cat, a thought bubble would appear above her head with a question mark floating inside.

I bend down and pet the top of her head. "She's not here any-more," I say, and my cat makes a strange sad chittering sound. "Well, she's dead," I say. My cat chitters again.

The imaginary question mark does not, even in my imagination, vanish.

•

A confession: I still cannot think of a way to *not* interpret the death of the nurse's fish as a sign.

On the drive home from my presurgical testing, I found myself sandwiched between two semitrucks transporting coffins. I called my mother to tell her. "I'm on my way back from getting my tests done and I swear to *God*, I shit you *not*, I am stuck between two trucks hauling coffins."

"Put the phone down before you end up in one of those coffins," she said.

No matter how many times I look, on no website is there advice in regard to explaining death to a cat.

In some situations, there exists no story, no possible way to explain.

127

As it turns out, I am not very good at having a hysterectomy.

When people asked how I was doing, I never knew how to respond. I'd say that I was doing well and in the breathless way one says one's doing well after, say, a five-mile uphill hike, or after an AP Calculus exam, or after one has looked up from one's unfinished french fries and Frosty to see one's ex and that ex's current girlfriend, staring at the double cheeseburgers while holding hands. I sent texts like this to the few friends I'd told about the surgery: *I slept forever and am about to take a shower and wash my hair, after which I will put on non-disposable panties, a nightshirt, and knee socks.* The only positive thing about surgery, I added, is that these are considered accomplishments.

I cried for the first time ten days after surgery. It was impressive in its suddenness. It was the type of crying that begins not in awareness that one is about to cry but that one is crying, and in loud and ugly ways. The most logical route seemed to be to just go with it, so I did.

"Oh," my mother said, and then "Emmy" and then "oh" again. We were awkwardly hugging or she was awkwardly hugging me and I made sounds that weren't anywhere near words.

I didn't know what I was thinking until I finally managed to say it: "I don't think I expected this." Then I thought *oh* and *oh* again, because I was right. I kept talking and listened to myself as I did, since

I seemed to be making a great deal of sense. I was telling my mother that I knew I had to have a hysterectomy, but that's different than having a hysterectomy. I wasn't using the actual word, *hysterectomy*, just its replacement, *it*, perhaps because *it* could've been anything. *It* could've been another round of birth control pills, or wearing PajamaJeans, or refusing to ever wear non-PajamaJeans ever again.

"I know, Peanut," my mother said. "I know."

"There's no going back from here," I said. I had made a decision, but the appointment and the surgery date came so fast, and the time in between was so full of paperwork and blood tests and Band-Aids and laxatives that I either had not had time to actually think about it or I had convinced myself that I had not had enough time to actually think about it. Or, perhaps, I had thought about it—I just hadn't thought about its afterward.

"That might've been a good thing," my mother said. "And you have to go through this. You can't go around it. It's been ten days and you haven't even cried."

I wished that she was wrong. I wished that we as human beings had gotten much better at avoidance and had built a detour that could take me around instead of through. I wanted to sleep. I wanted to sleep and wake into a world that was easier to put into words, and therefore to understand.

128

THREE WEEKS AFTER MY HYSTERECTOMY, I WENT TO THE bathroom. I wiped. And there it was. A red blotch on the white field of the toilet paper. It took me a moment to get past the ritual of expected annoyance, to remember that there was no longer any good reason for that blood to be there. I didn't have a uterus, so I shouldn't have a period. I looked through my surgical instructions to see if I should contact a physician. They were unclear at best.

"It says to call if the bleeding is heavier than a period," I told my mother. "But wouldn't that be, like, a major emergency?"

My mother reminded me of an important distinction: the surgical instructions meant *a* period, not *my* periods. "Keep an eye on it," she said, and so I decided to just ignore it for as long as I could.

And then I could no longer ignore it.

I was almost asleep. I was listening to the sounds of my parents, deep-sleep breathing and snoring on an air mattress in the living room. My mother had been staying with me since my surgery, and my father had driven the seven hours from Birmingham to south Georgia for Father's Day. I listened to the sounds of my cats, deep-sleep breathing and snoring on the bottom of my bed. I tried to sleep. I prayed for sleep. But instead of sleep, I felt this strange feeling, a new pain in my lower back. It started off like a dull ache, like a knee overused on an Exercycle, but soon the dull sharpened. The ache twisted into a tearing. I stayed in bed and tried to think of anything—how to conjugate French verbs, how to make the alphabet in sign language, how to write a sestina—except pain.

I could only think about pain.

I could only think about how strange this pain felt, as if something deep, down below the base of my spine, was being ripped apart.

And then I felt something wet.

Oh my God, I thought. *Oh my God, I am peeing myself. I am just lying here, actively peeing myself.* I told myself there could be no other explanation. I told myself that I was too close to sleep to get up. And anyway, I had on a hospital-issued sanitary pad, just in case; disgusting as that may be, it'd safely catch the pee. I didn't want to get out of bed because I didn't want to know what'd happen to that rip-apart pain if I stood. I shifted to the left, then the right. I felt more liquid. Something about it sent an alarm to my brain. Soon my whole body rang with it, as if my entire body shouted: *Get out of bed, get to the bathroom, get to the bathroom.* And then I was out of the bed and rushing into the bathroom. I was turning on the lights. I was pulling down my underwear and looking down at the floor.

It wasn't pee. It was blood.

It was blood, and it was everywhere. In the pad, on my underwear, spread in thick circles over my thighs, in drops on the bathroom floor. I managed to sit on the toilet and blood rushed out. I watched the crimson of it, overflowing the inelegant mattress of a Kotex from the box I got when I left the hospital, like a graduation gift, along with a pink plastic bowl in case I needed to puke on the car ride home. I wiped and looked at the paper: crimson. I looked at my hand, the fingernails clipped so I wouldn't scratch cuts into my skin when the pain medicine made me itch: crimson, dark in a border around the cuticles. I was staring. I was blank. I was not thinking. I was very calmly calling for my mother, who half-woke from her half sleep and called back, "What?" I was so calm. I was so calm that she didn't at first recognize the notes of emergency in my voice. We'd had a nice night of watching *Dateline*, drinking bourbon. We've had a nice night of celebrating a successful surgery and the successful life I now had the chance of living. My mother was annoyed, I could tell, and so I tried to be very calm as I told her, "I'm bleeding."

"What?" she called back, more awake and less annoyed, and I told her to come here. I told her it was bad. I heard the rustle of sheets and the air mattress squeaking and then she was in the bathroom with me, looking at the blood. She might have said *Emmy*. She might have said *shit*. She might have said *what happened*, or *what did you do*, or *what did you do that you weren't supposed to do*. I do know that she said, "I'm dizzy."

Within minutes, all the lights in my duplex were on. My father looked for the surgical papers while my mother and I wiped up blood with toilet paper and white washcloths. I told her I'd gotten white washcloths because they could be bleached.

"Good idea," she said. "Hand me the phone, then get in that bed." I handed her the phone. I got in that bed.

My mother called the number listed on my papers and reached one of the oncologist's endless assortment of aides and assistants. He seemed very confused. He seemed very young—a medical student who had a bow tie and the face of an eighth grader—and this was the first time he'd dealt with postsurgical bleeding. He asked how much blood and my mother handed me the phone, mouthing *I'm dizzy* before she laid down in bed beside me.

I told him a lot of blood. I used the word *gush*. "The toilet bowl was full of it," I said.

"Do you mean that there was a little blood," he said, as if offering a correction, "and when it hit water, it turned the water pink?"

"I mean there was a lot of blood," I said. "I mean so much blood that the water looked red. Not pink."

"Hm," he said, and I heard the click of his fingers against laptop keys. I thought, *He is totally googling this*. I thought, *You might be hemorrhaging under the care of an eighth grader who has to ask Google what to do in case of a hemorrhage*. I wondered, almost casually, if I was going to die.

The medical student asked if I could wait it out. "*Can* I wait it out?" I asked him. I resented him for making me the keeper of this decision. He said that if the bleeding stopped, then yes. He said I could just wait and see.

And so the medical student and my mother and I decided to wait and see. My mother stayed in bed beside me, trying to not be dizzy. I stayed in the bed beside my mother, trying to not be dying. I watched the ceiling fan spin and spin. I imagined myself on the ceiling, watching my body, pale-faced and perspiring. I looked at myself from the ceiling until it felt too much as if I was spinning along with the fan.

"Maybe don't look at the fan," I told my mother. "Maybe the fan is dizzy."

"What?" She held her hand over her eyes. "Stop being dramatic," she said. "Don't talk crazy. If you're going to the hospital, you don't need to talk crazy." This seemed like good advice, so I closed my eyes so my ceiling self couldn't look down at me, in the bed. I couldn't stop feeling, though. I couldn't stop feeling the rip-apart pain. The violence of it, decisive as any moment from which there is no turning back.

I bled for two hours before we decided I needed to go to the hospital. I couldn't stop apologizing. I apologized to my mother for ruining another pair of panties, for getting blood on my sheets, for not having the wherewithal to call the numbers on my discharge papers myself. I apologized to my mother for apologizing.

On the phone, I apologized to another one of the oncologist's endless assortment of assistants, who told me not to be sorry but to get to the nearest ER. He apologized in turn. He didn't know what to do: he was an hour's drive away, and at the rate I was bleeding, the drive could be dangerous. The nearest emergency room was one block away, so I didn't have to apologize about that. I did apologize to my father, who was driving, who was frightened, and who, I said, had to be having, like, the *worst* Father's Day ever.

I apologized to the intake nurse, who was clearly pregnant, who stood on one side of me with a male nurse on the other side of me. They half-walked, half-pulled me to the bathroom, and then the intake nurse walked into the bathroom with me.

"I've just got to see it so I know what you're talking about when you're talking about blood," she said. I pulled down my pants and my underwear and there it was, a gush.

"Yikes," she said.

"I'm so sorry," I said.

I apologized to the tech who took the urine sample I handed to him. "It's all blood," I told him. "I'm sorry. I tried to keep it out but there was just no way."

I apologized to the male nurse who tried to take my blood. "They're just very bad veins," I told him. "They roll out of the way."

"I can see that," he said. And then he held on to my upper arm and thumped my hand with his thumb, as hard as he could. When that didn't work, he used his fist, slamming my hand so hard that my body shook the bed.

"I'm sorry," I said. "I'm sorry, please stop, I'm sorry."

"I am very good at this," he said. "I can do this to babies and they never even cry."

"I'm sorry. I just need a break."

He threw the rubber strip on my chest, the needles on the equipment tray. I apologized to the back of his feet, to the back of his hand, which he raised and waved as if to say, *Don't try to speak to me, don't even speak.*

I was weak. I apologized to my parents for my weakness, for just having had too much. They nodded and mumbled and I turned my face away. I didn't want them to see me cry. I was too ashamed.

Six days later, I could still see them: five purple circles on my upper arm, arranged in a pattern immediately recognizable as the fingers on the nurse's left hand.

129

"I DON'T KNOW IF I CAN DO THIS," THE EMERGENCY ROOM doctor said, "but if you'll be patient with me, I'll try." I'd been in the emergency room for two hours. I nodded. I told her I'd be patient.

The this to which the ER doctor referred was a full vaginal exam, speculum and all. She wasn't a gynecologist, and she was terrified. All her calls asking for a gynecologist in the area to come in had failed. Finally, in confused desperation, she called the numbers on my discharge papers. She spoke to a different resident, who reassured her: this was fine, I was fine, the surgery went just fine. There was no need to put me in an ambulance so that I could be closer if not to the surgeon then to his students. And so the oncologist's student told the ER doctor how to perform a vaginal exam under my circumstances.

It is actually decidedly unclear if my surgery did indeed go just fine. No one involved in my hysterectomy told the story the same way.

From the pathologist's report, I know that my ovaries were peppered with several kinds of cysts, some large and hemorrhagic and filled with blood. My fibroid was larger than the uterus itself. The uterus itself was swollen and covered with adhesions. The endometrial lining had broken through and grown in the muscle of the uterus.

In other words, I know what the surgeon found. I have no idea how he found it, or what he did with what he found.

My recovery room postop conversation was unlike conversations I'd had after all my previous surgeries. There were no photographs documenting the pink landscape inside of my pelvis, no images of internal landmarks before and after endometriosis was excised, no mention of the adhesions that glued my uterus down against the pelvic wall.

In the hospital, some of the oncologist's students said my uterus and ovaries were unremarkable. Some reported a fibroid of minimal size; some compared it to a large orange or a small grapefruit. In their notes on the surgical file I finally obtained, I found no mention of cysts, of endometriosis, of the careful exploration of my pelvic region and peritoneum that necessitated the skills of an oncologist in the first place. Around 5:00 a.m., a student informed the nurse that the surgeon had insisted that my catheter be removed. Around 7:00 a.m., another student asked the nurse why she had disobeyed the surgeon's orders and removed the catheter.

The nurses—I know, I remember—shook their heads, turned their hands into fists, and hid them behind their backs. The nurses—I know, I remember—apologized.

After three years had passed, I finally managed to get my complete operative report. I thought that the thick wad of surgical records would tell the story I knew the oncologist was supposed to tell me. And they did tell me part of the story: every time nurses entered my room during my hospital stay, every pill they gave me, every time they asked me to breathe into a plastic tube to move a ball up in the air. The nurses lifted the side rails on my bed so that I wouldn't roll out. They noted that I lost an estimated 55 ccs of blood during the surgery, that my urine output was 150 ccs. From these records, I know all the peripheral facts orbiting the surgery itself. What I don't know is what happened during the surgery itself—moment by moment, scalpel cut by scalpel cut—or who made it happen.

I know this information should be in my records. And I know

where that information should be in my records. Here is what that page says:

PAGES MISSING

There are six other pages that say, simply: NO DATA FOR THIS REPORT.

This is how the oncologist's student suggested that ER doctor examine me: upside down, strapped to a hospital bed tilted at a forty-five-degree angle so that I wouldn't slide off.

"Oh," I said.

"Are you kidding me?" my mother asked. My father sat very straight in his chair. I could almost hear his teeth grinding.

"I'm sorry," I said to my father and his teeth, to my mother and her *are you kidding me* voice, to the ER doctors and her hands, which felt along the bottom of my hospital bed to find the levers that would flip my body upside down.

"We will be as careful as humanly possible," the doctor said, "and if I think I'm doing damage or I'm hurting her too much, I'll stop." My parents, tight-lipped, teeth grinding, nodded in agreement. I didn't nod in agreement because no one expected me to. I was in the hospital, which, I'd learned, was a place where my consent never mattered.

My parents shuffled out of the room and the doctor pulled the curtain between us. It looked and sounded like a mint green shower curtain from the seventies, whooshing and rattling its way across a metal pole. Then it was just the doctor and my body and me. There was an emergency room technician in the room, too, whose job was to drop off medicines and deal with various tubes and bandages, and since she had never seen someone who had just had a total hysterectomy bleed excessively, she asked the emergency room physician if she could stay and watch, as if my body were there to put on a show, to perform, whether I wanted that or not. The emergency room physician gave her assent, and then remembered that the vagina in question was not hers but mine.

"If it's okay with the patient, of course." She tilted her head to the side and looked over my legs at me. I didn't know how to do anything but agree.

The upside-down position, the ER doctor said, would help her see the cuff without having to use the speculum aggressively, which could damage the cuff even more than she suspected it'd been damaged.

"What's a cuff?" the technician asked, and I said, "Good question." A cuff, the doctor explained, was what they made in a female human body after removing its cervix, so that all the other nonreproductive human organs in the pelvis, such as intestines both large and small, did not fall out.

"Ew," the technician said.

"Agreed," I said.

"Think of it like a sock," the ER doctor said, "like an inside-out tube sock," so both I and, I'm assuming, the technician thought of it like a sock. The sock I pictured was pink and sort of strange and the kind of thing that would be very uncomfortable to wear, which was exactly what my bleeding cuff felt like to me. The nurse and doctor found the right levers and then my feet were above my head, my head angled downward. I wondered if it was possible to calculate the slope of the line on which my body lay. I wondered if my parents could hear any of this, so I angled my head until I could see under the curtain. I saw their shoes there, tapping the linoleum. I closed my eyes.

The doctor told me to take a few deep breaths. To get ready. I opened my eyes. She told me to open my legs, then peered between them. I looked at her looking at the most private parts of me. Except they weren't exactly private, anymore. They were more like a struggling settlement centered in a battle between hospital and hospital, doctor and doctor, student and teacher. I closed my eyes again.

"It looks as if your cuff is intact, so I'm going to try to examine it." She asked the technician to hand her a pediatric speculum. The technician obeyed. "Deep breath again, Emily," the doctor said. "Deep breath." I felt the edges of the speculum and then I felt a kind of pain beyond fire, a bolt that breaks the body into its electricities. Maybe I gasped, or maybe I almost-screamed, or maybe I made no sound but was betrayed by some unconscious motion of my body, or maybe the doctor realized there was no way to insert the speculum without ripping something apart. All I remember is that she dropped the speculum back on the instrument tray, where it clattered and clanged. I remember. She put her hands up in the air.

"I can't do it, I'm sorry," she said. "They're just going to have to do this themselves, because I can't do this to you. I'm sorry."

130

THE FIRST ER DOCTOR SENT ME HOME WITH MORE HOSPITAL pads, more nausea pills, more antibiotics for the UTI they suspected because my catheter had been removed too soon. She told me to call the oncologist's students if I started to bleed again, to tell them I was in the car and headed their way. "Don't ask them if you should go. Just go."

"He needs to see his own damn patients," I overheard her telling a nurse as she walked out of the room.

"They said they close things up by making something that looks like a tube sock," I said to my mother when we were alone. I used the voice I use to make it clear that I think something's totally disgusting.

"Well, they can't just leave it flapping open," she said, and I imagined a door taking advantage of its hinges. I imagined a plastic pet flap and an indecisive cat. I tried to imagine the inside of my body and failed. I sent Deena a text to tell her I'd been in the emergency room. I told her that they tried to examine my cuff.

What the fuck is a cuff, Deena texted back, so I texted the thing about the sock.

Like Lamb Chop, she responded.

Exactly, I texted back.

Hours after I was discharged from the first ER, I sat with my mother in the ER an hour's drive away, bleeding. I couldn't stop in-my-head singing that Shari Lewis song with no end, the one that goes on and on, my friends. And everywhere I looked, everything—the walls I knew to be aqua, the white paper pulled over the examining table, my mother, the doorway, the fluorescent light—was gray. I lay on the hospital table with a wad of paper towels tucked underneath me while a resident inserted a speculum to examine my cuff. She jerked the speculum back and forth. She was not gentle. She was confused. She couldn't stop herself from making *hmmmm* noises. I couldn't stop myself from saying, "That doesn't sound too encouraging," and my mother couldn't stop herself from shaking her head and raising her eyebrows in agreement with me.

The resident pursed the left side of her mouth. "The cuff seems to be intact," she said. She shook her head a little bit more. "I have a plan, but I'm going to need your help to go through with it."

This was the resident's plan: She would find and use the largest speculum possible. She would push this speculum as far into my vagina as possible. She'd spread it apart as far as it would go. She'd take small sticks of silver nitrate and cauterize both ends of the cuff. In other words, she would burn the tissue in my newly formed cuff as thoroughly as she could in the hopes of closing off the wound.

"You have got to be kidding me," my mother said.

"But you just said that the cuff was intact," I said. "You said there was no wound."

She didn't pause to explain what she meant. Instead, she continued to explain my part in her plan: "This is going to hurt. It's going to be tremendously painful. But once I get started, I have to finish. I cannot stop. You have to be still and be patient, and you can't move or scream."

I wasn't looking at her anymore. I was looking at the top of her head, at the place where the light's fluorescence hit the black of her hair and made it blue. I was thinking it was a beautiful sight, like a neon halo. I was thinking, *What choice do I have but to just lie here?*

What point would there be in trying to scream? And so I told her I'd be patient. I promised to be a good patient.

She promised pain medicine and Phenergan. She'd make sure I was comfortable. She left to confer with her attending about the plan to which I was forced to agree.

131

THE HOSPITAL RECORDS FROM MY SECOND EMERGENCY ROOM visit seem totally optimistic.

They also refer to a woman who is totally not me.

The woman in the report is thirty-two, not thirty-three.

She has an O- blood type, not A+.

She is allergic to Nicorette but not aspirin.

She had only three prior laparoscopies for endometriosis, which she's had only since the age of seventeen.

Her last laparoscopy was in 2009, not in 2010.

She's never had a small bowel repair.

Her recovery period, according to a resident, "was unremarkable."

The bleeding she noticed was slight—just some spotting on toilet paper and a dime-size clot.

Upon examination of her pelvis, the resident found no "obvious active bleeding," though "areas of adherent clot were cleared." The next sentence, however, mentions "a small area of oozing" on both sides of her cuff, both of which were cauterized with silver nitrate.

The report is not clear as to what, exactly, oozed, or from where, or why.

The report doesn't explain how the resident determined the oozing wasn't blood or why she would cauterize the oozing if it wasn't blood.

The report—of course—does make it clear that this me-not-me patient is "doing extremely well from a postoperative standpoint."

132

A WEEK LATER, MY MOTHER DROVE ME TO MY ONE-MONTH-postsurgery check-up. The oncologist determined that I was completely healed. I was still bleeding. When I mentioned that, he flipped to his resident's notes for my second ER visit, which, I later found out, state that "no bleeding was noted at the end."

Bleeding was, in fact, noted at—and after—the end.

After the resident burned the tissue tying together both sides of my cuff, she told me to lie on the table until I was discharged. My blood pressure kept diving downward. I worked diligently at not passing out. A nurse appeared with pills and a paper cup of water as well as my discharge papers. She put her arm around me and helped me, slowly, make my way off the table upright. I had an hour-long car ride in front of me, so I asked to use the restroom and for a hospital pad, just in case. The nurse and my mother helped me to the bathroom. I was standing on the other side of a closed door, awkwardly pulling down my underwear, when it happened again.

Blood.

There were five or so feet between me and the toilet. I tried to run, but those five or so feet still were spotted with blood. I wiped and looked and then a woman who might have been me said, "Oh God."

In the center of my hand sat a blood clot. The size of my open palm.

I slid it onto a wad of paper towels then folded the towels over to cover the clot. I don't remember how I made it to the bathroom door. I don't remember how I opened it, or how long I stood there, looking out and up and down the hall and saying, "I need some help, I'm sorry, please."

The nurse who'd given me the pills and the water and the discharge papers looked up and then, when she saw my face, ran. I showed her the clot.

"Oh God," she said, so I showed her the bathroom, the blood on the tile, on the toilet, in the toilet. She called for my mother, who'd been signing papers. She called for someone to please page the resident who'd seen me, and immediately. "She's going to want to see this," the nurse said. "She's going to have to pack the wound."

We'd just finished cleaning the blood off the tiles when the call from the resident came through. A little spotting was common after a hysterectomy, she said. She had discharged me. She refused to admit me again. There was absolutely no need, she said, for me to be seen.

I looked at the nurse and she looked at me. She handed me a box of hospital Kotex.

"Well," she said, "I guess that means you're free."

"The bleeding is fine," the oncologist said at my postsurgical check-up. "A little spotting is common. Just wear a panty liner for the time being."

"I'm not just spotting, though. And a panty liner is nowhere near enough."

"I've had a hysterectomy," my mother said. "I didn't bleed like that."

He made a little *pshew* noise. He made a little flick with his hand. "Sure, she's been bleeding, and she may bleed again. It should taper off eventually." He put my file in my hand and told me to follow the blue stripe on the tile to the checkout window, then hand my file to the receptionist.

I followed the blue stripe on the tile. My mother followed behind me, a hand close to my back in case I fainted. It seemed equally possible, at all times, that I would move into another step or that I would pass out. I handed my file to the receptionist. I saw my mother's hand reach out, as if by reflex, as if she knew that it was equally possible that I'd hand the receptionist my file or that I'd drop it.

"Looks like he's released you completely," she said. "From now on, call your regular gynecologist if you need anything."

I couldn't look at her, so I looked at the corner of the glass above her and nodded. I was too angry, but I was also ashamed.

133

After my hysterectomy, I became, for the first time in my life, very good at being angry and not so good at being sad.

I wrote cruel responses to posts by not-quite-in-real-life friends on Facebook. I took Diet Cokes from the refrigerator, tapped the silver over the spout, and bent the tab back and forth, saying a letter of the alphabet until the tab broke off. Mary taught me how to do that when we were in seventh grade. She told me the last letter you reached before the tab broke was the first letter of your future husband's name. The tab always stopped on the letter *D*. I thought, *Daniel? Darien? Damien?* I checked Facebook for responses to my mean comments. I wanted to fight. I wanted to keep fighting. I never wanted to fight again.

I deleted my comments, response or not. I deleted the not-quite-in-real-life friends from my Facebook friends list. I worried about hurting my not-quite-in-real-life friends while taking off my clothes and waiting for the water in the shower to heat. I worried about myself while washing and conditioning my body and my hair. I said, "What is wrong with you," out loud to the hair dryer, the cosmetic applicator sponge, the eyeliner, my reflection, myself. I tried to think about something else while putting on lip gloss. I made mental checklists while zipping my dress pants. I told myself to (1) be calm and (2) stay off Facebook to keep myself calm. Then I'd drive to work and I'd always be late and yelling at the slow driver of the slow car in front of me, "For Christ's sake, I hate this fucking town and I hate everything and everyone in it."

When I said I hated everything in this fucking town, that included me.

I decided to start cooking. I decided to quit my job. I didn't quit my job. I did quit cooking. I looked at photographs of my grammar school friends and hated them for their families. I looked at photographs of my grammar school enemies and I hated them even more for their families. I started praying. I stopped believing in God. I kept praying anyway.

134

"LET ME ASK YOU SOMETHING," MY MOTHER ASKED ME A FEW weeks after surgery. "Are you upset because you will never have children or are you upset because you *can't* have children?"

"Hm," I said, and looked at my coffee cup, which looked back like a blank black eye, which is how I felt.

"Do you know what I mean?" my mother asked, and even though I didn't, I told her I did. I looked past the coffee cup to the coffee table. On top of it sat a stack of small fabric hexagons. I kept telling myself that I was going to make them into a quilt, but I really just made them into a task: their making, their matching, their color-coding, from hope white to dead yellow to sky black. I thought. I tried to imagine my home with a child, and just like every time I tried, someone else's child appeared, toddler-pink-cheeked, a visitor holding out banana bread wrapped in tinfoil and tied with a bow. Then I tried to imagine myself wanting a child. I tried to imagine the conversation with my husband—invisible-faced, a shadow in the corner of my mental picture's frame—in which I said, *It's time for us to talk about perhaps having a child.*

"Well," I said to my mother, still looking at all the points of fabric, all the lines waiting to be joined and sewn, "I think it's that there's just no going back."

•

Two months after my hysterectomy, I walked through the summer heat to the university's printing and postal services facility located in a back room in the main dining commons building. Except I didn't walk, per se. I walked only approximately. I struggled, I could say, except *struggle* implies a sense of dignity seriously diminished by my failing deodorant, by the sweat beading itself into a glittering mustache above my lipstickless lips. I heaved myself forward, clomp by clomp. I lurched. I galumphed. I ogred. I was suddenly aware of the experience of my own body as nothing like my own body, as something closer to a collection of sodden embarrassments. I could no longer see myself as I existed or as I had previously existed. I could no longer see myself as my self. *When did I become this*, I wondered, *when did my legs become two reluctant animals who would rather do any of the world's elses besides carry my body to the printing and postal services facility?*

I slipped into a back hallway in the main dining commons. I knew that, especially during the summer, that particular hallway would be relatively empty, which meant I would not have to see myself being seen. I would not have to raise my chin and smile and hello. I would not have to focus both on the effort of chin raising and smiling and helloing and of walking the two animals that were my legs at the same time. The full-blast late-summer Deep South air conditioner raised prickles on my skin but did not stop my sweating, which had at this point slicked my hair against the back of my neck.

I tried to forget about it: the bad animals that were my legs, the sweat beading and slicking my body. I tried to forget about everything. I opened and walked through the door to the printing and postal services facility. I walked to the counter, looking down and focusing very intently on my feet, on the black-and-white spectator oxfords my mother called rah rahs because she wore them as a cheerleader in high school. I'd double-knotted them before leaving the house but they were still half unlaced. I begged them not to trip me, focusing intently, trying to control the feet inside of them until they acted like feet. *Be feet*, I thought at them, *be feet, be feet, be feet.* And then I was at the counter.

I took a deep breath and released the breath, deeply. I prepared myself to look up. I arranged the features of my face into an expression I hoped would indicate that I was a capable and intelligent woman, that I was capable and intelligent and together-gathered enough to bear the responsibility of educating young adults gathered in classroom groups of fifteen to thirty. I recognized but tried to hide from myself an awareness of sweat settled and pooling in the small of my back. I recognized but tried to hide an awareness of heat spreading its red across my cheeks. I raised my head. I reminded my body to try to be normal. I reminded myself that I was here in this facility as a professor in higher education. I smiled and my lips stuck dry against my teeth. A woman with blond hair immaculately lacquered into an immaculate French twist stood before me in a buttoned twinset. She smiled and her Clinique-pinked lips followed her directions perfectly.

"Can I help you?" she asked in a highly moss-in-the-trees Savannah accent. I attempted to smile more broadly. I attempted to stand in such a way as to suggest I too owned a twinset or at least knew where one would purchase such a thing.

"I'm here to pick up the course packet for my class. Under Bolden." I pulled the paperwork from the front pocket of my purse and slid it across the counter to her, cursing myself for folding it into fourths as she smoothed out the creases, cursing her for not being the hungover summer employee I had expected.

She held the paperwork by the top right corner and nodded. "Coming right up," she said, and I both admired and hated her for the ease of her response.

When her back turned, I fanned myself with my hand and then pulled my collar forward repeatedly, fanning air onto my chest and down my dress. I looked down and saw my white bra now sweat-dampened to gray. I wiped my forehead with the back of my hand and then looked with horror at the streak of sweat and CoverGirl foundation left behind. The woman returned, still perfectly blond and perfectly smiling, a cardboard document box in her hands. She let it fall on the counter with a thud and though I tried to remain politely void of expression, I felt grateful for the brief burst of air.

She asked me if I wanted to examine the course packet for correctness. I did not want to examine the course packet for correctness. I did not at that moment give even the slightest shit about the course packet's correctness. I wanted to grab the packet in its cardboard box and force my feet to run out of the printing and postal services facility, through the back hallway and the parking lot to my car, where an air conditioner and a glove compartment full of fast-food drive-through napkins perfect for mopping up sweat awaited me. But I felt as though there were a social contract I'd signed when I signed my contract for a tenure-track position, that I would break that contract, disappointing her and the gravity of my position, if I did not at least feign a great concern for the correctness of my course materials.

I removed the box's cardboard top. I lifted the course packet from the bottom of the box. I leaned over, preparing to flip through its photocopied pages. And then it happened. A drop of sweat fell from my nose, hitting the cardboard box top with an audible plop. I looked down at it in horror, a small circle seeping at its edges into the cardboard, a singularity of all the shame my body carried around as it carried me around. I couldn't stop looking at it, this gray circle of evidence. And then it was as if my tongue took the side of my body and decided that yes, this was the moment to give up control, this was the moment to unsecret the secrets I had worked so hard to keep.

"I'm so sorry," I said. "It's so hot outside and I just had a hysterectomy and it didn't go well."

I expected the blond woman's perfect to crack. I expected her lips to curl into a Clinique-pink grimace of disgust. Instead, she softened, her immaculate eyebrows falling into an expression of sympathy.

"Oh, sweetie," she said. "I'm so sorry." She leaned forward and I realized that she smelled like perfume, like good perfume, like actual perfume and not cologne or body spray. She glanced to the left and to the right, checking, I realized, to make sure that we were still the only two people in the printing and postal services facility. Still, when she spoke, she lowered her voice to a rumble just above a whisper. "I sweat like a hog when I had mine," she said. "It took me forever to get my hormones straight."

I could not stop my mouth from falling open. At the same time, I could not make my mouth obey enough to respond, so I just nodded.

She shook her head. "It's a rough time. It's a rough time for sure, sweetie. But you're so young. Do you mind my asking how old you are?"

I asked myself if I minded. Strangely and for reasons I did not understand, I answered that I did not mind, I did not mind her asking at all. "I just turned thirty-three," I said.

She made a *whew* sound in response, drawing it out into several syllables, moving the pitch of her voice up and down and up again, the way one does in response to a story that seems too absurd not to be true. "Lord, you are young," she said. "Are you married? Did you have babies? I mean, I don't mean to pry."

I tried to decide if she did, indeed, mean to pry. I didn't have an answer for that, though I did notice that she didn't ask if I minded her asking. I decided to ask myself if I minded anyway. I answered: I minded slightly more than when she asked how old I was, but surprisingly, I found I didn't mind a lot. And so I told her no. And then my mouth started its work again, started telling her everything, everything: I didn't because I couldn't, I had this fibroid, it was bigger than the uterus itself, and I had endometriosis, too, and everything inside was bound together and there was so much pain, so much pain, so much I could no longer take. I could not at that moment tell why I'd decided to tell her. Perhaps because she was a stranger. Perhaps because she'd asked. Perhaps because a different social contract was now in play, and according to this contract, if I wasn't married and didn't have children and agreed to allow a surgeon to remove the organs that would allow me to have a child, it required an explanation.

When my mouth had stopped its talking, I realized I was sweating even more. I realized that I was worried about her reaction, that I wanted to run again, and far, before her perfectly Clinqued face revealed her feelings of disgust. Then I realized that she was nodding in a way that indicated that she understood, and deeply. She was nodding in a way that indicated the sympathy of a shared experience.

"Sweetheart, be glad it's all gone." She leaned forward even further, all good perfume and hair spray, breath freshened by sweet mint gum. "The day I had my hysterectomy was the happiest day of my life. I sat up and thought to myself, *Whew, that's over.* I just sat up and finally felt free." And then it happened: her mouth, her beautifully Dramatically Different™ lipsticked mouth, opened and her voice carried words the way mine had, as if her mind had no part in this, as if her mind couldn't stop it if it wanted to, the way her mouth was letting out words. She had gotten married—and divorced—and was lucky enough to have one daughter, but no one knew how. She had fibroids too, three of them, the size of oranges, and who in the world thought to compare them to fruit anyway?

And she also had endometriosis, and when they got in there, it was everywhere: her bladder, her bowel, everywhere, and she bled so much that they gave her iron shots to cure her anemia, and she loved her daughter but sometimes wished for her sake that she had been a boy because she'd passed all her problems down to her, except her daughter's were worse, she'd had too many fibroids to count and anemia that once sent her to the emergency room. And as she spoke I nodded and nodded. I thought to myself at first, *What is this, a competition?* I thought to myself at first that this was her way of telling me that my problems were nothing compared to her and her daughter's problems, that this was her way of telling me that she thought I should've held on longer. And then I realized that I was the one who was telling myself this. I wasn't used to this kind of conversation, this kind of war story, this kind of speaking openly about the secrets our bodies had hidden inside of themselves. I started to wonder how many women, how many perfectly perfumed and hair-sprayed women, how many perfect women in perfectly buttoned twinsets lived inside of bodies that had so betrayed them.

She kept talking and I kept nodding, and then her mouth reached the end of the words it had to make. She sighed and made the *whew* sound again. "I don't know," she said. "I just felt so free. Do you feel free?"

I looked her in the eye. They were beautiful green eyes, Savannah-live-oak eyes, with four shades of purple Clinique All About Shadow™ so perfectly applied that, had she not told me, I'd never would've suspected how exhausted she'd been, how doubled-over-pained she'd been, for so much of her life.

I nodded. I closed my eyes and nodded.

"Yes," I said, "I know exactly what you mean. I just feel freed."

THE SHIP OF THESEUS

135

ONE AUGUST MORNING MY CAT MOVED AROUND THE FOYER, making a face. I said "What?" and she kept making the face. Then I remembered: her ball. I threw it and she chased it, periscope-tailed. "I felt like I was in one of those depression commercials," I told my mother that night. "The ones where the woman makes her dog sad." I told her that I thought I'd been doing well. I thought I had been doing very, very well.

That day, my mother had lunch with her friend, the nurse, for the first time since my surgery. "I showed her about how big your fibroid was," and I saw her, at the Olive Garden, making a larger-than-an-orange circle from her fingers over the endless salad and breadsticks. She asked her friend if I could have lasted through a pregnancy, if I even conceived a baby at all.

"She said no." My mother used her very sure and serious voice. "She says you couldn't have gotten pregnant, and if you did, you would've miscarried. Or bled out."

And though I didn't know, though I don't know, I said, "I know." My voice also sounded sure and serious, and in my mind, I added what her friend said to my story. It fit so naturally. I told myself that one day I wouldn't even remember that part of the story not being there.

136

SINCE MY TOTAL HYSTERECTOMY, I'VE EXPERIENCED REGULAR vaginal bleeding. I experienced vaginal bleeding so regularly, in fact, that I began charting it. After a few months, these charts confirmed my suspicions: the bleeding happens on a monthly cycle, exactly like a menstrual cycle. Sometimes the bleeding is light. Sometimes the bleeding is heavy. Sometimes the bleeding makes me so dizzy that I have to lean against a wall. Once, I fell off a stool. And with the bleeding comes pain: the same kind of pain I felt in bed the night I went to the emergency room, that same kind of ripping-apart pain.

Eight years after my hysterectomy, I had an MRI to check for diverticulitis. While the radiologist saw no sign of that, he did note an incidental finding: degenerative disc disease, resulting in a herniated disc and, I later discovered, severe damage to the sciatic nerve. When I told my mother on the phone, I couldn't help but cry.

"They know what it is," I said. "They actually know what it is. There's a name. And they know how to treat it."

I wonder if this has always been the answer, the reason why my leg refused to feel or walk or stand.

Later, I followed a suspicion and googled *Lupron degenerative disc disease*. And there it was, the first result: an article about women who were prescribed Lupron to stop early puberty, women who now, in their twenties, reported symptoms and diagnoses of conditions that typically affect much older women, such as osteoporosis, cracked bones, cracked teeth, arthritis, and degenerative disc disease.

A week after I found out about the herniated disc, I saw a gynecologist for my annual Pap smear. The appointment was quick and efficient. At the end, the gynecologist leaned against the door and looked at me, still sitting on the examining table, awkwardly trying to hold the back of my paper robe shut.

"Well," he said, "I still think it's what I've thought it was, which is that they left part of an ovary with endometriosis in it behind." I stared at him. I made myself blink. That was the first time I had heard this information. I did not say that. I did not say anything. I knew better, by that point.

"Sorry we can't do anything about it. At least you're not in horrendous pain anymore."

Then the gynecologist was gone, and all that was left was for me to hurry back into my clothes and go home.

An answer is not the same as a solution. I know that by now too.

I have gotten very good at being angry.

Friends and former classmates post photos of their pregnant bellies, sometimes years after their babies are born. In captions and comments, they describe their admiration for their own bodies. They use words like *fierce* and *strong*. They use words like *miracle*. I dutifully click digital hearts to digitally like each photo. I pause. I wonder. What must it feel like, to see your body as fierce and strong, as a miracle? I wonder and don't wonder if in some small and incomparable way, I should see my body in the same way. Because it survived. Even when I didn't want it to. It survived.

When I told a friend of mine I was still bleeding, that I was still having periods, she said, "HOW IS THAT POSSIBLE," and I said, "I DONT KNOW," and both of us said it just like that, in all caps with no punctuation marks. "It's like RAIN FROM NO SKY," she said, which might be more accurate than anything any physician, emergency or otherwise, ever told me about my body.

Every semester, at least once, my students and I would get into a conversation about the word *ambiguous*. The conversation would quickly slip into the kind of fight people have when they're arguing about something that they don't entirely understand simply because that something cannot be entirely understood by anyone. The word *ambiguous* is a good example of this because the word itself is ambiguous. In the everyday way of using the word, *ambiguous* can mean "kind of vague." But in the less-everyday way of using the word, it can mean "containing a great many meanings as totally equally and at the very same time true." Both definitions are true, and both definitions are infuriating.

If there was one major theme in what the catechism taught me about holiness and human bodies, it is this: in order to be truly holy, a body must be truly ambiguous. It must be like Mary's body, which was with child and without intimate knowledge of man at the same time. It must be like Jesus's body, which was mortal and human but, at the same time, immortal and godly. It must dwell in two states of being—the possible and the impossible—at the very same time.

When my own body became ambiguous—when it was in

medically induced menopause while still in its teens, when endometriosis persisted and spread while targeted with treatments every doctor swore would work, when it experienced periodic bleeding after
going through menopause—I should have known what was coming.
I should have prepared myself for doubt. I should have known how
many men would doubt, would demand proof, would have to put
their hands inside of my wounds.

137

WHEN I WAS IN COLLEGE, I LEARNED ABOUT THE SHIP OF Theseus, also known as Theseus's Paradox.

This is Theseus's Paradox: the Athenian king Theseus won a great battle while sailing a specific ship. Because its story was important, the Athenians thought this ship was important, too, so they decided to preserve it. As the wood got older, it did what everything and everyone does with age, which is to say it decayed. The Athenians removed the decayed wooden boards and replaced them with new wooden boards. And philosophers really like to talk about this ship and about these boards because it gives them a way to talk about this question: *If the base of the ship they tried so hard to preserve rotted away, if the old boards are removed and replaced with new boards, can it be said to be the same ship, or is it now a different ship entirely?*

I ask myself: Is the body I walk and talk and move around in now the same as my body before surgery?

If I still have uterine tissue, could it still be said that I have a uterus?

If I still bleed at periodic intervals, do I still have periods?

If there are no medical solutions, can these be called medical problems?

I tell myself the story—or, at least, the details that I know. I remember. I don't remember. I shape. I shift. I order and reorder. I tell and retell. I wonder: Will these pieces coalesce and connect, will they rise to climax and fall into place, into peace? Will I ever put my body and my self back together, if they were even together in the first place?

I wonder if it's even possible, if a cohesive story is even a place in which a body and its soul can be. If instead the time we spend living is more like floating in a sea in which there's no such thing as sinking or swimming, in which the only choice is to be moved by its waves and to learn how to surrender to that movement, to look through the water for the light even when we feel we're drowning.

Notes

5   *the same as the blood on the Shroud of Turin*: Kelly P. Kearse, "Blood on the Shroud of Turin: An Immunological Review," Shroud of Turin Website, 2012, shroud.com/pdfs/kearse.pdf.

13   *That's what happened to Sister Lúcia of Fátima*: For a description of beliefs about Lúcia of Fátima and her message about modesty, see Fr. Shenan J. Boquet, "The Message of Fatima, the Family, and the Crisis of Modesty," Human Life International, October 13, 2017, hli.org/2017/10/message-fatima-family-crisis-modesty.

37   *According to Ronald E. Batt's* A History of Endometriosis: Ronald E. Batt, *A History of Endometriosis* (London: Springer-Verlag, 2011).

42   *I was reading chapter 3 of* The Interpretation of Dreams: Sigmund Freud, *The Interpretation of Dreams*, trans. A. A. Brill (Digireads.com Publishing, 2017).

80   *On July 3, 1980, the United States Conference of Catholic Bishops*: Information about tubal ligation in Catholic hospitals is from the United States Conference of Catholic Bishops' *Statement on Tubal Ligation* released on July 3, 1980, and described in *Contraception, Sterilization, & Abortion*, accessed January 16, 2022, usccb.org/issues-and-action/marriage-and-family/natural-family-planning/catholic-teaching/upload/Contraception-2.pdf.

80   *Only in 2019 did the Vatican clarify*: Amy Littlefield, "Vatican Approves Hysterectomies If Your Uterus Isn't 'Suitable for Procreation'," *Rewire News Group*, January 9, 2019, rewirenewsgroup

.com/article/2019/01/09/vatican-approves-hysterectomies
-if-your-uterus-isnt-suitable-for-procreation.

80   *There were still approximately 2 million oocytes*: Eric Nagourney,
"What Happened to All Those Eggs?" *The New York Times*,
February 1, 2013, nytimes.com/2013/02/01/booming/womens
-eggs-diminish-with-age.html.

84   *Though endometriosis has been mentioned in medical texts for
4,000 years*: Camran Nezhat, Farr Nezhat, and Ceana Nezhat,
"Endometriosis: ancient disease, ancient treatments," *Fertility
and Sterility* 98, no. 6 Supplement (December 2012): S1–62,
fertstert.org/article/S0015-0282(12)01955-3/fulltext.

84   *promoted by a doctor named John Sampson*: For more information about John Sampson, see Adi E. Dastur and P. D. Tank,
"John A Sampson and the origins of Endometriosis," *The Journal of Obstetrics and Gynecology of India* 60, no. 4 (July/August
2010), 299–300, ncbi.nlm.nih.gov/pmc/articles/PMC3394535
/pdf/13224_2010_Article_46.pdf.

84   *He called this process retrograde menstruation*: "9 Endometriosis Facts Our Doctors Want You to Know," Fertility Answers,
accessed January 19, 2020, fertilityanswers.com/9-facts-our
-doctors-want-you-to-know-about-endometriosis.

84   *Mercury is in retrograde 24.657 percent of the year*: Calculation
based on information in Kerry Ward, "Your Mercury in retrograde 2022 survival guide: Meaning, dates and everything you
need to know," *Cosmopolitan*, January 11, 2022, cosmopolitan
.com/uk/horoscopes/a34629295/mercury-retrograde-meaning
-dates-guide.

84   *according to a Gallup poll*: Linda Lyons, "Paranormal Beliefs Come
(Super)Naturally to Some," Gallup, November 1, 2005, news
.gallup.com/poll/19558/paranormal-beliefs-come-supernaturally
-some.aspx.

93   *Alfred Kinsey and his team of sexuality researchers*: "The

Kinsey Scale," Kinsey Institute, accessed November 19, 2021, kinseyinstitute.org/research/publications/kinsey-scale.php.

93   *Kinsey, himself bisexual*: According to the Legacy Project, biographies published after Kinsey's death showed that he was actively bisexual. Victor Salvo, "Dr. Alfred Kinsey - Inductee," Legacy Project, accessed November 19, 2021, legacyprojectchicago.org/person/alfred-kinsey.

105   *On April 9, 1985, the FDA approved a drug for the treatment of prostate cancer*: For more information about Lupron's initial approval, see the FDA Drug Approvals and Databases. "New Drug Application (NDA): 019010," FDA Drug Approvals and Databases, last modified December 10, 2018, accessdata.fda.gov/scripts/cder/daf/index.cfm?event=overview.process&ApplNo=019010.

106   *where it finds the gonadotropin-releasing hormone receptor*: For a brief explanation of how GnRH agonists and antagonists work, see the NIH's National Cancer Institute website. "GnRH antagonist," National Cancer Institute, accessed November 17, 2021, cancer.gov/publications/dictionaries/cancer-terms/def/gnrh-antagonist. For more detailed information, check out ScienceDirect's overview of GnRH agonists and antagonists. "GnRH Antagonists," Science Direct, accessed November 17, 2021, sciencedirect.com/topics/neuroscience/gnrh-antagonists.

106   *On January 26, 1989, the FDA approved a new form of Lupron*: For more information about the approval of Lupron for use in women, see the FDA Drug Approvals and Databases. "New Drug Application (NDA): 019732," FDA Drug Approvals and Databases, last modified March 4, 2019, accessdata.fda.gov/scripts/cder/daf/index.cfm?event=overview.process&ApplNo=019732.

106   *More than 7 million American women have been diagnosed with endometriosis*: Lena Felton, "The House just doubled funding

for endometriosis research, thanks to its second-youngest member," *The Lily*, July 31, 2020, thelily.com/the-house-just-doubled-funding-for-endometriosis-research-thanks-to-its-second-youngest-member.

111   *A 2015 study found that 74 percent of women*: Hanna Howard, "Most Straight Girls Are Actually Also Attracted to Other Girls," *Teen Vogue*, November 6, 2015, teenvogue.com/story/straight-girl-bisexuality.

127   *In a letter written not long after he was married*: Rainer Maria Rilke, *Letters of Rainer Maria Rilke, 1899–1902*, as quoted in note 19 of *Letters to a Young Poet*, translated with an introduction and commentary by Reginald Snell (Mineola, NY: Dover Publications, 2002) 45.

129   *However, only 43 percent of women bleed*: Kate Moriarty, "The Truth About Virginity in College," *Her Campus*, March 11, 2015, hercampus.com/wellness/truth-about-virginity-college.

133   *Of the hymen, Alfred Kinsey wrote*: Kinsey's comments about the hymen appear in his 1950 suggestions on the manuscript of a new edition of Abraham Stone and Hannah Mayer Stone's *A Marriage Manual: A Practical Guide-Book to Sex and Marriage*. Wardell B. Pomeroy, *Dr. Kinsey and the Institute for Sex Research* (New Haven: Yale University Press, 1982), 164.

139   *According to the Endometriosis Foundation of America*: "What Is Endometriosis?" Endometriosis Foundation of America, accessed January 15, 2022, endofound.org/endometriosis.

140   *An Australian study found*: For more information about the Australian study and other research, see Omar T. Sims et al., "Stigma and Endometriosis: A Brief Overview and Recommendations to Improve Psychosocial Well-Being and Diagnostic Delay," *International Journal of Environmental Research and Public Health* 18, no.15 (August 2021), ncbi.nlm.nih.gov/pmc/articles/PMC8346066.

140   *A 2006 study showed*: Carolina Lorençatto et al., "Depression in women with endometriosis with and without chronic pelvic pain," *Acta Obstetricia et Gynecologica Scandinavica* 85, no. 1 (2006): 88–92, pubmed.ncbi.nlm.nih.gov/16521687.

141   *Later, this was found to be untrue, as hysteria also happened in male bodies*: According to Elaine Showalter's *Hystories*, Charcot opened a ward for male hysterics in 1882. Elaine Showalter, *Hystories* (New York: Columbia University Press, 1997). The narrator of the semi-autobiographical *The Notebooks of Malte Laurids Brigge*, published in 1910, seeks treatment at the Salpêtrière Hospital, presumably in the ward for male hysterics.

146   *A "visuel," a seer*: Carlos Henrique Ferreira Camargo et al., "Jean-Martin Charcot's Influence on Career of Sigmund Freud, and the Influence of This Meeting for the Brazilian Medicine," *Revista Brasileira de Neurologia* 54, no. 2 (2018):40–46, docs.bvsalud.org/biblioref/2018/07/907032/revista542v4-artigo6.pdf.

155   *According to a 2017* Kaiser Health News *article*: Christina Jewett, "Women Fear Drug They Used To Halt Puberty Led To Health Problems," *Kaiser Health News*, February 2, 2017, khn.org/news/women-fear-drug-they-used-to-halt-puberty-led-to-health-problems.

155   *According to Lupron's own prescribing information*: *Highlights of Prescribing Information*, AbbVie, Inc., last modified March 2020, rxabbvie.com/pdf/lupron3month11_25mg.pdf.

155   *According to a KTNV Las Vegas news report*: Darcy Spears, "More women come forward with complaints about Lupron side effects," KTNV Las Vegas, last modified February 12, 2019, ktnv.com/news/investigations/more-women-come-forward-with-complaints-about-lupron-side-effects.

156   *According to the prescribing information on the Lupron Depot website*: "Lupron Depot for Endometriosis," Lupron Depot, last modified April 2021, luprongyn.com/lupron-for-endometriosis.

163   *Four months later, on October 20, 2010*: While the FDA's October 2010 warning letter to Sanofi-Aventis is no longer available on the FDA website, you can find a description on the *Monthly Prescribing Reference*'s online archives. "GnRH antagonists labeling updated to include diabetes and cardiovascular risk," *Monthly Prescribing Reference*, October 21, 2010, empr .com/safety-alerts-and-recalls/gnrh-agonists-labeling-updated -to-include-diabetes-and-cardiovascular-risk/article/181413.

163   *In their May 2010 news release*: "FDA Drug Safety Communication: Update to Ongoing Safety Review of GnRH Agonists and Notification to Manufacturers of GnRH Agonists to Add New Safety Information to Labeling Regarding Increased Risk of Diabetes and Certain Cardiovascular Diseases," FDA, last modified December 13, 2017, fda.gov/drugs/drug -safety-and-availability/fda-drug-safety-communication -update-ongoing-safety-review-gnrh-agonists-and-notification. For more information about adverse drug reports and Lupron's side effects, see the Lupron Victims Hub at lupronvictimshub.com.

164   *An article in* The Journal of Minimally Invasive Gynecology: J. Cory Barnett, MD, et al., "Laparoscopic positioning and nerve injuries," *The Journal of Minimally Invasive Gynecology* 14, no. 5 (September 1, 2007): 664–72, jmig.org/article /S1553-4650(07)00160-4/references.

164   *A 2000 study found*: Mark A. Warner, MD, et al.,"Lower Extremity Neuropathies Associated with Lithotomy Positions," *Anesthesiology* 93 (October 2000): 938–42, pubs.asahq.org /anesthesiology/article/93/4/938/38610/Lower-Extremity -Neuropathies-Associated-with.

168   *the contortions that Charcot named* attitudes passionnelles: Georges Didi-Huberman, *Invention of Hysteria: Charcot and the Photographic Iconography of the Salpêtrière*, trans. Alisa Hartz (Cambridge, MA: MIT Press, 2003), 115.

181   *He later wrote a bedroom prayer*: Saint Alphonsus Liguori, "Good Night Prayer," Novena Prayer, May 25, 2020, novenaprayer .com/2020/05/25/good-night-prayer-by-saint-alphonsus-liguori -1696-1787.

183   *The shutter opens: Mlle Bairet, black-clad and brass-buttoned*: This passage describes a four-photo series taken at the Salpêtrière Hospital by Londe in 1885 titled "Mlle Bairet, electrostimulation" found in Albert Londe, *Photo Poche No 82* (Paris: Actes Sud, 1999), image 16.

185   *In order to become a doctor, a person instead swears to this*: Charles W. Eliot, ed., "The Oath of Hippocrates," *The Harvard Classics* (New York: P. F. Collier & Son, 1910) 38:3.

185   *In October 2001, TAP Pharmaceutical Products*: A full list of charges against TAP Pharmaceutical Products can be found on the Department of Justice's website. Department of Justice, "TAP Pharmaceutical Products Inc. and Seven Others Charged with Health Care Crimes; Company Agrees to Pay $875 Million to Settle Charges," news release #513, October 3, 2001, justice.gov/archive/opa/pr/2001/October/513civ.htm.

186   *A third charge: according to a 2001* New York Times *article by Melody Petersen*: Melody Petersen, "2 Drug Makers to Pay $875 Million to Settle Fraud Case," *The New York Times*, October 4, 2001, nytimes.com/2001/10/04/business/2-drug-makers-to -pay-875-million-to-settle-fraud-case.html.

191   *According to a 2009 article published in the* Journal of Gynecological Endoscopy and Surgery: S. Krishnakumar and P. Tambe, "Entry Complications in Laparoscopic Surgery," *Journal of Gynecological Endoscopy and Surgery* 1, no. 1 (January–June 2009): 4–11, ncbi.nlm.nih.gov/pmc/articles/PMC3304260.

191   *On the* Golf Digest *website, Dustin Johnson writes*: Dustin Johnson, "Dustin Johnson: How To Hit A Flop Shot," *Golf Digest*, June 19, 2016, golfdigest.com/story/dustin-johnson-how-to-hit-a-flop-shot.

194   *In a 2018 paper published in the* Journal of Pediatric & Adolescent Gynecology: Jenny Sadler Gallagher et al., "Long-Term Effects of Gonadotropin-Releasing Hormone Agonists and Add-Back in Adolescent Endometriosis," *Journal of Pediatric & Adolescent Gynecology* 31, no. 4 (August 2018): 376–81, ncbi.nlm .nih.gov/pmc/articles/PMC5997553.

194   *They mention the discussion forums and petitions that proliferate online*: The Lupron Victims Hub maintains a database of Lupron-related lawsuits that can be accessed here: lupronvictimshub.com/lawsuits.html.

209   *she sneezes and sneezes and cannot stop*: There have been several stories about girls who can't stop sneezing that received widespread media coverage, including Brooke Owens (2007), Katelyn Thornley (2015), and Lauren Johnson (2009), whose story I describe. The segment in question is Yunji De Neis and Sarah Netter, "Achoo! Lauren Johnson Can't Stop Sneezing," ABC News, November 11, 2009, abcnews.go.com/GMA/OnCall /lauren-johnson-girl-stop-sneezing/story?id=9051534.

213   *A Reddit user posts a version of her video*: Though the video is no longer available, see post by rickyisawesome, "12 Year old Lauren Johnson can't stop sneezing. Here is a montage of her problem from The Today Show at 117 Sneezes Per Minute." Reddit, November 16, 2009, reddit.com/r/videos/comments /a4z95/12_year_old_lauren_johnson_cant_stop_sneezing.

213   *On a CNN segment, an expert discusses her symptoms*: The CNN segment aired on November 13, 2009. Dr. Sanjay Gupta discusses Lauren Johnson's case. Newsstube, "Lauren Johnson Sneezing girl," video, 4:09, November 13, 2009, youtube.com /watch?v=agq6ClZSodk.

218   *In a 2006 segment on NPR's* Weekend Edition: Linda Wertheimer, "Ancient Sneezing: A Gift from the Gods," May

27, 2006, in *Weekend Edition*, npr.org/templates/story/story
.php?storyId=5435812.

219   *It takes a year for doctors to give the girl a name and a reason*:
Mike Celizic, "Bless you! Girl who kept sneezing has stopped,"
TODAY, March 11, 2010, today.com/health/bless-you-girl-who
-kept-sneezing-has-stopped-1C9399358; "Girl Who Sneezes
12,000 Times a Day Gets Official Diagnosis," Fox News, last
modified January 14, 2015, foxnews.com/story/girl-who-sneezes
-12000-times-a-day-gets-official-diagnosis.

240   *In Greek mythology, Cassandra was a princess of Troy*: Laura
A. Shamas, "Understanding the Myth: Why Cassandra
Must Not Be Silenced," *On The Issues Magazine*, July 13, 2011,
ontheissuesmagazine.com/2011summer/cafe2/article/163.

247   *If mathematics is "rightly viewed," Bertrand Russell writes*: Bertrand Russell, "The Study of Mathematics," in *Mysticism and
Logic, and Other Essays* (New York: Longmans, Green and Co.,
1919), 60.

271   *a fertility drug "used to mature the eggs and trigger their release
at the time of ovulation"*: "Female infertility," Mayo Clinic, accessed June 2, 2021, mayoclinic.org/diseases-conditions/female
-infertility/diagnosis-treatment/drc-20354313.

279   *On the front page of the Asexual Visibility and Education Network's website*: Though this note has since been deleted, one can
see this note and a discussion about it on the Asexual Visibility
and Education Network's "Questions about Asexuality" fo-
rum, accessed June 3, 2021, asexuality.org/en/topic/16333-note.

284   *But there's a value missing from the scale*: "Creating the scale,"
Kinsey Institute, accessed November 19, 2021, kinseyinstitute
.org/research/publications/kinsey-scale.php.

292   *According to Circle Surrogacy, a Boston-based surrogacy agency*:
"One All-Inclusive Cost Program," Circle Surrogacy, accessed

January 4, 2022, circlesurrogacy.com/parents/how-it-works/surrogacy-cost.

292   *According to WebMD, women under the age of thirty-five have only a 37.6 percent chance*: "Infertility and In Vitro Fertilization," WebMD, August 1, 2021, accessed January 16, 2022, webmd.com/infertility-and-reproduction/guide/in-vitro-fertilization.

293   *In an interview with NPR, University of Southern California fertility specialist Richard Paulson*: Patti Neighmond, "Women Can Freeze Their Eggs For The Future, But At A Cost," in *All Things Considered*, October 16, 2014, npr.org/sections/health-shots/2014/10/16/356727823/freezing-a-womans-eggs-can-be-emotionally-and-financially-costly.

293   *One of the drugs used to improve egg production in IVF cycles*: For more about the use of Lupron in IVF, see "Lupron (Leuprolide)," Fertility Center of Oregon, accessed January 16, 2022, fertilitycenteroforegon.com/lupron-leuprolide.

References

The information about hysteria and the Salpêtrière was synthesized from the following sources. The girl's story is imagined, but based on these source materials:

Breuer, Josef, and Sigmund Freud. *Studies on Hysteria*. Translated and edited by James Strachey. New York: Basic Books, 2000.

Carson, Anne. "The Gender of Sound." In *Glass, Irony and God*, pp. 119–42. New York: New Directions, 1995.

Cixous, Hélène, and Catherine Clément. *The Newly Born Woman*. Translated by Betsy Wing. Minneapolis: University of Minnesota Press, 1986.

Didi-Huberman, Georges. *Invention of Hysteria: Charcot and the Photographic Iconography of the Salpêtrière*. Translated by Alisa Hartz. Cambridge, MA: MIT Press, 2003.

Freud, Sigmund. *Dora: An Analysis of a Case of Hysteria*. New York: Touchstone, 1997.

Kumar, David R., BS; Florence Aslinia, MD; Steven H. Yale, MD; and Joseph J. Mazza, MD. "Jean-Martin Charcot: The Father of Neurology." *Clinical Medicine & Research* 9, no. 1 (March 2011): 46–49, clinmedres.org/content/9/1/46.

Kushner, Irving. "The Salpêtrière Hospital in Paris and its role in the beginnings of modern rheumatology." *The Journal of Rheumatology* 38, no. 9 (September 2011), 1990–93, jrheum.org/content/38/9/1990.

Londe, Albert. *Photo Poche No 82*. Paris: Actes Sud, 1999.

McCarren, Felicia. *Dance Pathologies: Performance, Poetics, Medicine.* Redwood City, CA: Stanford University Press, 1998.

Micale, Mark S. *Approaching Hysteria: Disease and Its Interpretations.* Princeton: Princeton University Press, 1995.

Mitchell, Juliet. *Mad Men and Medusas: Reclaiming Hysteria and the Effect of Sibling Relationships on the Human Condition.* London: Penguin Press, 2000.

Showalter, Elaine. *The Female Malady: Women, Madness and English Culture, 1830–1980.* New York: Pantheon, 1986.

Showalter, Elaine. *Hystories: Hysterical Epidemics and Modern Media.* New York: Columbia University Press, 1997.

Vincentian Encyclopedia. "The September Massacres in Paris and Versailles." Updated May 4, 2007. famvin.org/wiki/The_September _Massacres_in_Paris_and_Versailles.

My notes from Dr. Michael Robinson's Ibsen class, University of East Anglia, fall 2000; Dr. Jo Catling's Poetry and Painting: Rilke and Modernism class, University of East Anglia, spring 2001; Dr. Marvin Frankel's The Talking Cure class, Sarah Lawrence College, fall 2001–spring 2002; and my independent research projects in courses taught by Esther Podemski (Drawing, Sarah Lawrence College, fall 2001–spring 2002) and Kate Knapp Johnson (senior thesis, Sarah Lawrence College, fall 2001–spring 2002).

Acknowledgments

Thank you to the following journals, where portions of this manuscript appeared in an earlier form:

- "Glossolalia," *Blossombones: The Freud Issue* (Summer 2010).
- "Precipitation," *Yalobusha Review* 16 (2011).
- "About the Human Hymen Membrane (Disambiguation)," *The Rumpus* (March 5, 2014).
- "About My Tenth Year as a Human Being," *Prime Number Magazine* 61 (October–December 2014). Reprinted in *Prime Number Magazine, Editors' Selections: Volume 4.* Edited by Clifford Garstang, Valerie Nieman, Jon Chopan, and Brandon D. Shuler (Winston-Salem, NC: Press 53, 2014).
- "Counting the Lovelies," *Tupelo Quarterly* 6 (February 27, 2015).
- "My Only Carriage: On Naming a Nameless Disability," *The Toast* (August 12, 2015).
- "Good Girl," *Panoply* 2 (Winter 2015/2016).
- "Up a Steep and Very Narrow Stairway," *StoryQuarterly* 50 (2017).
- "Patient History (Small Bowel Puncture)," *District Lit* (June 30, 2017).
- "Strand Tests," *Tupelo Quarterly* 14 (February 2018).

For a book that is, at its core, about enduring pain, the process of bringing it into the world has been one of the greatest joys of my life.

I am so grateful for my team at Soft Skull Press, with special thanks to Jordan Koluch and Samm Saxby. Thanks to Nicole Caputo for this perfect cover and to Wah-Ming Chang for her design work. I am especially grateful for my editor, Sarah Lyn Rogers, who *saw* the book and understood it in a way I'd only ever dreamed of having someone see it. I couldn't have dreamed of a better, wiser, more brilliant editor for this book, and there aren't enough words to express my gratitude and appreciation for you, for your kindness, your generosity, and your talent. Thank you, from the bottom of my heart.

Endless gratitude to Cassie Mannes Murray, my agent at Triangle House Literary, for believing in this strange beast of a book when it was a messy ghost of its current self, and for helping it find the shape it needed to say what it needed to say. Thank you also for keeping the faith when my own faith faltered, for all the all-caps messages and the absolutely perfect GIFs. You are a force of good in this world and I am so lucky to know you.

I first started following the thread of hysteria in women's history as an undergraduate at Sarah Lawrence College, and I owe a great deal of gratitude to the professors who guided my research and writing and encouraged a multidisciplinary approach. Special thanks to Kate Knapp Johnson and Esther Podemski for their wisdom, guidance, and inspiration.

My gratitude to Gina for being the best best friend anyone could ask for. I promise I'll let you play the bongos during one of my readings someday.

I wrote the first pieces of this book in 2008. Since then, I've been lucky to have so many supportive, wonderful friends and colleagues who helped me make it, day by day, both through my struggles with my own body and with my struggle to wrestle this story into a form that made sense on the page. I'm especially grateful to Hannah Dela Cruz Abrams, Chantel Acevedo, Julianna Baggott, Holly Barbaccia, Karen Bender, Katt Blackwell-Starnes, Wendy Brenner,

Dustin Brookshire, Garrard Conley, Kristin Czarnecki, Kristina Marie Darling, Danielle DeTiberus, Zoe Howard Sally J. Johnson, Hallie Johnston, Nicole K., Katie Dobosz Kenney, Catherine Lawrence (Req), Rebecca Lee, Allie Marini, Sarah Messer, Brooke Middlebrook, Laurel Mills, Jessica Nastal, Rachel Nix, Jared Rizzi, Ashley Roach-Freiman, Mike Scalise, Alina Stefanescu, and Brigitte Wallinger-Schorn. Special thanks to Ross White and to the members of the Grind community for helping me to write and keep writing.

For my former students, who showed me what it means to write with integrity and bravery. You taught me more than I could ever have taught you.

For the doctors who listened and helped.

My deepest gratitude to the National Endowment for the Arts and the Alabama State Council on the Arts, whose generous grants supported the writing of the poems that became the doorway through which I entered this memoir.

Finally, for my parents. I don't know how I was lucky enough to have two parents who aren't just incredible parents but who are amazing human beings as well. It's impossible for me to articulate just how very grateful I am for you each and every day—words will never suffice. Thank you for always being there and always lifting me up (sometimes literally). This book is for you, with all my love. Thank you.

Special thanks to Brigitte Wallinger-Schorn for her translation of the Rilke quote that serves as an epigraph.

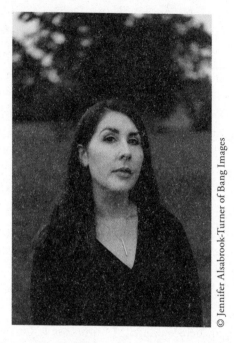

© Jennifer Alsabrook-Turner of Bang Images

EMMA BOLDEN is the author of *House Is an Enigma*, *medi(t)ations*, and *Maleficae*. She is the recipient of a National Endowment for the Arts Literary Fellowship, and her work has appeared in *The Norton Introduction to Literature*, *The Best American Poetry*, *The Best Small Fictions*, and journals including *Mississippi Review*, *Seneca Review*, *StoryQuarterly*, *Prairie Schooner*, *TriQuarterly*, and *Shenandoah*. She is the associate editor in chief for *Tupelo Quarterly*.